The Medical Interview Coach

Claire Teresa Lundy

The Medical Interview Coach

A Practical Approach for Healthcare Professionals

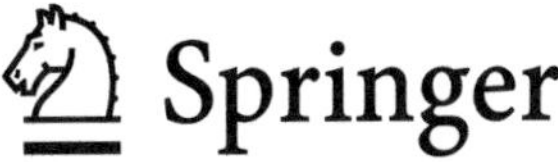 Springer

Claire Teresa Lundy
Consultant Paediatric Neurodisability, Accredited Coach
Health and Social Care Leadership Centre
Belfast, UK

ISBN 978-3-031-16320-3   ISBN 978-3-031-16321-0   (eBook)
https://doi.org/10.1007/978-3-031-16321-0

This Springer imprint is published by the registered company Springer Nature
Switzerland AG
The registered company address is: Gewerbestrasse 11, 6330 Cham, Switzerland

Preface

An interview is an opportunity to showcase your abilities, to share your knowledge and enthusiasm. Daunting? Maybe…

Using a coach approach as part of your interview preparation encourages personalised, confident answers. Coaching is used throughout many industries as part of workplace personal development. Using open questions, coaches support participants to have a deeper look at challenges in the workplace and develop their own tailored solutions. Coaches can also assist with a supportive approach to changing career direction, leadership coaching and executive coaching for senior leaders. In the sporting world, coaches are well recognised as helping athletes improve performance.

This interview primer is your personal 'interview coach'. The coaching questions in each chapter guide you to a better understanding of how to condense your experience and describe your skills in response to interview questions.

Preparing for your interview using the *The Medical Interview Coach* as a workbook will enable you to deliver clear, confident, eloquent answers which demonstrate your unique skillset, improving your chance of success at the interview!

Belfast, UK   Claire Teresa Lundy

Introduction: The Coach Approach to Interview Preparation

Interviewing for a new position as a medical professional should be an opportunity to share your enthusiasm and knowledge; however, for many people 'the interview' seems daunting and it's a struggle to condense years of experience into coherent answers that not only score points but convey clinical abilities and personal leadership style.

What Is the 'Coach Approach'?

The Medical Interview Coach is a practical guide which offers a structured 'coaching approach' to your interview preparation. Coaching is used throughout many industries and is best recognised in the sporting world. Coaches help athletes develop an understanding of their capability, solve challenges through training and ultimately this enhances performance. In other industries, coaches support individuals and teams to improve personal and team performance. Coaches may not be experts in the particular field but will bring skill and expertise in supporting their clients through the use of open questions and personal analysis. This technique can help the client identify goals, understand their work environment more fully, realise opportunities that exist and support the development of solutions to workplace challenges. Coaches also support career development through interview coaching, leadership development coaching and executive coaching. *The Medical Interview Coach* chapters will support you by working through different areas of healthcare practice using coaching questions to reflect on your experience and training. The questions will help you to identify your areas of strength and focus on how to highlight your unique skillset. Using this innovative 'coach approach' ensures that your answers are individual and targeted. The use of templates will help you structure your preparation and the sample questions bring opportunities to develop your answers.

The Medical Interview Coach will help introduce or consolidate your understanding of some of the language and terminology used in modern health care. These should not be seen as 'buzzwords'. Rather they help encapsulate important concepts and point to the fundamental basis of these ideas. The language and philosophy of an idea are usually closely intertwined. Demonstrating a working knowledge of commonly used terms is important when applying for a healthcare role.

The book also includes practical tips on analysing advertisements in advance so that you are off to a head start and highlights hot topics that will help you demonstrate your relevant knowledge. The 'My Notes' and 'Coach Approach' sections provide you with summary pages, as you work your way through each chapter. This unique coach approach to medical interview preparation will ensure you deliver personalised, relevant answers with a clear and engaging structure. Using this book will ensure the interview panel meet the real you and importantly, allow you to confidently demonstrate your passion for health care.

How to Use 'The Medical Interview Coach'

Giving yourself as much time as possible to prepare for an interview is obviously going to be helpful! *The Medical Interview Coach* will provide a 'workbook' style structure for your preparation with chapters providing an introductory topic overview followed by structured reflective exercises.

Ideally your preparation for a new permanent medical role such as a consultant or primary care physician should begin in the year you finish specialist training as it will be an opportunity to identify any outstanding training needs and address these. If you are thinking of applying for a specialty doctor role or a new role within your organisation, the same approach is relevant, as soon as you identify the opportunity take time to look at what the role requires and if you have the requisite training and skill set. There is guidance on how to work through an application, prepare for a pre-interview visit and undertake a video interview. The chapters provide a structured approach to reviewing your training and experience through the eyes of a potential employer rather than a training committee or a clinical supervisor.

If you have less time or are applying for an additional role such as a clinical specialty lead, quality improvement lead or department head, the chapters can be used as active interview preparation in the weeks before the interview. They provide structured reflections in the 'Coach Approach' sections and sample questions to practice.

Practising your answers with friends and colleagues is one of the most helpful things you can do. You can also try recording your answers and listening to your responses. Many people take the same approach as they did to exam preparation, writing out notes and preparing flash cards. An interview is different! The panel wants to be able to understand your approach to health care through your spoken answers, the best way to deliver confident, clearly articulated answers is to practice, practice and practice some more!

Contents

Practical Tips for Preparing Your Job Application Form

1

Everyone knows they should prepare well in advance for an important interview but the reality of busy working lives means few people actually do this!

You may have identified a hospital or medical unit where a vacancy is coming up or you are coming to the end of specialist training. During the months before the interview you will likely be working so setting aside some time on a regular basis for your preparation will help you feel less overwhelmed and anxious in the weeks before an interview.

As soon as you think you are going to look for a new role, or you are coming towards the end of your professional specialist training you should prepare your Curriculum Vitae (CV)/Resume and think about future interviews. You might wonder how to go about this when the role has not even been advertised, but it is easier than you might think! Check out similar jobs in other institutions; what skills and competencies were they looking for? Focus on the *essential* and *desirable* criteria. Make a list and cross-check this against your qualifications and credentials. If you know where you would like to work, look at currently advertised roles in that organisation, and start to identify key criteria that they look for in applications. This preparation will allow you plenty of time to start drafting out your application or Curriculum Vitae / Resume as well as identify areas that you need to develop or courses you need to attend in order to fulfil the job specification.

© The Author(s), under exclusive license to Springer Nature Switzerland AG 2022

C. T. Lundy, *The Medical Interview Coach*,
https://doi.org/10.1007/978-3-031-16321-0_1

1.1   The Advertisement

Most medical interviews are *competency based,* in this type of interview the questions are structured to allow clear scores of ability and competency in relation to specific skills outlined in the job description. Technical professional roles such as medical and surgical posts will require the panel to ascertain that you have the skills required to undertake the day-to-day work of the role, for example an Emergency Medicine doctor will need to be able to confidently explain their approach to the management of a major trauma call, a Histopathologist may need to describe their training and expertise in the analysis of surgical specimens including their approach to reporting and benchmarking with agreed standards. Each successful part of the answer allows the panel to award 'points' to the candidate.

Increasingly healthcare organisations are starting to incorporate *values-based* interview questions. These questions can explore how you are likely to behave in the workplace. Organisations recognise the importance of workplace culture and its impact on patient safety and employee well-being. Values-based questions allow the panel to see your approach to clinical leadership, your ability to work well with colleagues and to get a sense of your personal style of delivering patient care. Organisations are interested in understanding if are you someone who will drive improvement and innovation alongside your team.

1.2   Quick Wins!

The job advertisement is your starting point to identify the *competencies* the role requires. It will usually highlight some additional information on the organisation such as their corporate *values* and their *core work*. These are useful ways to prepare for the questions that might come up in the interview. If specific competencies and skills are outlined they are likely to come up as part of a question

Table 1.1   Key facts about the organisation

• Mission statement
• Organisational values
• Size and structure
• Key points about the department—staff/size/areas of clinical activity/ research activity

or clinical scenario. If organisational values are clearly stated, you can start to consider scenarios when you demonstrated these values through your behaviour in the workplace. See Table 1.1.

1.3   Get Shortlisted

There are often contact details for clinicians and managers you can speak to in advance of a formal application so you can decide if the role will suit your skill set and get a feel for the organisation. It may also provide some insight into areas of practice they particularly value or wish to develop. This will ensure that you clearly document relevant skills on your application form. Sometimes a proportion of the 'points' in an interview are awarded to the application form. The shortlisting process generates a 'score' related to the essential and desirable criteria. It is critical that you adopt a structured and diligent approach to filling in the form. This chapter provides a systematic approach and coaches you through the process.

The advertisement should give clear information on deadlines for applications and may give an indicative interview date. Many interviews are now virtual so you will need to consider access to appropriate technology. There is usually a link to an online application process and some organisations may also ask for a CV and cover letter. You may need to ask for time off to prepare and attend the interview, make arrangements for this as soon as you can to avoid additional stress in the days before the interview.

1.4   Employer References

It is worth thinking about who you might approach to be a referee at this stage as most organisations will require at least two and sometimes three references for a medical role. It is expected that at least one of these references will come from your current employer. Ideally, the individuals should know you well and have knowledge of your training and clinical skills in the relevant area. It is courteous to ask permission to use them as a referee and give them time to prepare a reference, this avoids the unwelcome scenario where a reference is not forthcoming after you have been conditionally offered a post! You should provide them with a copy of your most up-to-date CV and relevant information such as any absences you may have had or breaks in employment as often references come in an online format which requires this information. It is also helpful to provide your referee with contact details if they need to check any details with you.

1.5   The Application Form

It is really important to get the basics right. Use a spell check! Have someone else read over the document for you to ensure you have not missed any significant errors. In this section, you will use a structured approach to identify how you meet the *essential* and *desirable* criteria and learn how to ensure you are shortlisted.

1.6   Employment Details, Examinations and Qualifications

Ensure that relevant employment dates are correct and that your personal information and contact details are clear. Triple check any parts of the application form that relate to the documentation of examinations or qualifications that are in the *essential* and *desirable* criteria. If you do not document these as required on the form you may not be shortlisted.

1.6.1   'Coach Approach'

Use the job specifications to check *essential* and *desirable* criteria in each section of the application form. Use this template to note how you meet the criteria. It can be helpful to use a timeline to get started, ask a friend to help! See Tables 1.2 and 1.3.

Ensure that you have covered all of the *essential* criteria and referenced any additional skills you have that meet the *desirable* criteria. Describe as clearly and comprehensively as you can how you meet the criteria as some candidates will be sifted out on a review of their application if they have put insufficient or scanty information. The application form may be 'scored' as part of the process for example 25% with the other 75% of points available at the interview. This means your application form is extremely important as it is not only a means of getting over the hurdle of shortlisting but it is the first part of your interview process.

Table 1.2 Essential criteria

• Examinations
• Specialist training/certifications
• Core technical skills
• Relevant professional courses
• Accreditations
• Quality improvement qualifications and key projects
• Audit/benchmarking
• Teamwork/personal development skills and qualifications
• Patient engagement and feedback
• Appraisal and revalidation
• Specialist societies/memberships
• Publications/presentations
• Awards

Table 1.3 Desirable criteria

• Examinations
• Specialist training/certifications
• Core technical skills
• Relevant professional courses
• Accreditations
• Quality improvement qualifications and key projects
• Audit/benchmarking
• Teamwork/personal development skills and qualifications
• Patient engagement and feedback
• Appraisal and revalidation
• Specialist societies/memberships
• Publications/presentations
• Awards
• Additional clinical skills/relevant qualifications

1.7   Qualifications

Be very clear about relevant dates of any qualifications and awarding institutions. You will generally be asked to provide copies of certificates when you attend an interview or when you are formally offered the position. It is a good idea to pull all this information together as soon as you start the application process in case you need to apply for copies of documents you have misplaced.

You will also be asked to confirm your accreditation and practice licensing, and document any significant issues that you have faced with respect to your practice. It is also important to ensure that you are in good standing in terms of subscription payment with any memberships that you will be referencing on your application, for example a Royal College or Specialist Society. If you undertake appraisal and revalidation ensure that you have documented your current status. Many healthcare jobs also require a driving license. You may be asked to note any criminal convictions.

1.8   Clinical Skills

The first section of the application form is often the outline of clinical skills required for the role. For example, if it is a consultant surgical post there may be specifications laid down about the particular area of surgical expertise required. As you start your preparation begin to think about your experience or expertise that you have which relates to the skills described as essential criteria. You can set out your training and qualifications in this area chronologically so that it is easy to shortlist. It may be more straightforward to list the most recent first as these are likely to be the most relevant. Ensure that you have mentioned all of the key areas that demonstrate how you meet the essential criteria. The next step is to look for desirable criteria in the same area and identify if you meet these specifications such as being able to offer a new technique or being able to train others in a similar area.

Other *essential criteria* tend to be around existing commitments that a department may have, such as particular techniques, education or expertise in research. It is important to be able to clearly describe during your interview and in any application form exactly how you meet the essential and any desirable criteria in these areas.

When describing clinical skills it is important to demonstrate on the application form that you are both competent and confident in the performing of particular practical procedures or skills that have been deemed *essential*. If you have undertaken a training course or have recognised exams in this area highlight this very clearly in the application.

1.9   Credentials and Qualifications

The job specification and application form will give you a clear description of essential qualifications needed for shortlisting, for example particular exams or accreditation with a professional organisation. Describe qualifications as clearly as possible. When you are in your interview make sure that you reference the *essen-*

tial criteria as part of your answers. If you have any *desirable* criteria such as additional exams, awards, qualifications or specialist experience in a particular field reference these criteria in your application form and CV.

1.10   Specialist Experience

Document your specialist credentials clearly including dates and awarding professional bodies. You may have acquired experience and training working in a clinical environment in another country. You will need to ensure that you demonstrate equivalence with respect to the *essential* criteria.

If you have something additional to offer and you can highlight that this meets both *essential* and *desirable* criteria describe this as clearly as possible using bullet points if necessary to demonstrate how you will bring additional expertise to the department. It is useful to also report the duration of any additional training, giving dates and institutions where you were employed and who supervised the post (Box 1.1).

> **Box 1.1 'Coach Approach'**
> What did you achieve in your time abroad? How long did you work there? Who was your supervisor?
> Describe the unit-what techniques did you learn, did you complete any qualifications?
> Was the approach to healthcare different? What did this mean for your training and healthcare practice?

1.11   Additional Skills

The application form may have a section which allows you to describe additional information such as projects you have undertaken, this can be a good opportunity to describe specialist technical skills, time management, project planning, awareness of stakeholder engagement, data management, teamwork, communication and financial planning. For example, describe an improvement project by including title, project aims and outcomes. When describing personal attributes it is useful to think about what is relevant to the position, for example highlighting any personal development that you have undertaken in areas such as communication skills, mentorship, patient safety training, research methodology or quality improvement.

It may also be helpful to highlight any feedback that you have received with regard to your personal attributes in the workplace such as approachability, ability to deliver on project deadlines and ability to work well within a team environment. If your work resulted in the team achieving an award or recognition in the organisation record the details and describe the benefit of the work (Box 1.2).

Box 1.2 'Coach Approach'
What workplace feedback have received recently?

- Colleagues
- Patients
- Supervisor
- Personal reflection
- Multisource workplace feedback/360
- Awards
- Applications

What did you learn about yourself and the service you provide? How did the feedback influence your approach to healthcare?

Use these reflections to consider ways to document your personal attributes in the additional information section.

Outline any additional areas of expertise that may bring value to the role. These may have been gained in work outside the health sector such as involvement in an outside charity or business that has helped you with time management and people management skills, highlight the institutions or companies involved and relevant dates. See Box 1.3.

Box 1.3 My Notes
- Recent project/research
- Aim
- Outcome
- Benefits for patients/staff
- Key skills
- Additional personal skills
- Other experience/expertise/qualifications

1.12   Research and Education

Research and education expertise can be key components of healthcare positions, particularly if the organisation is affiliated with a university. If you have a research degree it is important to be very clear about the dates and the institution that awarded the research qualification. In the application form, it is helpful to provide a short description of the work that you undertook and your key outcomes. If this work resulted in publications highlight these in chronological order starting with the most recent. A similar approach can be applied to presentations at conferences; international, national, and local.

Many healthcare roles have an educational aspect to them as it is expected that you will be able to support the training of others in your department. If you have additional qualifications or formal education training provide the awarding institution and the relevant dates on your application form.

Highlight particular skills clearly, for example having the ability to develop and deliver an online curriculum, experience of teaching using virtual ward rounds, simulation skills, problem-based learning, mentorship and educational supervision training. Describe any roles that you have such as designated educational or clinical supervisor or postgraduate lead in your specialty area.

If this is an area that you are hoping to develop and you are at an earlier stage in your career you can note that you are willing to take on additional responsibility and highlight any relevant training that you have undertaken to date and any positive feedback on training that you have been involved in. See Boxes 1.4 and 1.5 for preparation ideas

Box 1.4 'Coach Approach'
What makes you a qualified applicant in terms of research/educational experience?

How would you describe your research/educational training to a layperson?

Can you describe a timeline of your research career and what your key projects delivered?

Box 1.5 My Notes
- Research projects
- Research awards
- Education training
- Education Responsibilities

1.13   Innovation and Quality Improvement

The application may have a section on quality improvement, innovation and patient safety. Most organisations will have a specific approach to healthcare improvement and will be looking for candidates who can help achieve the organisational goals around safety and quality.

If you have been involved in quality improvement projects and have received training in this area it is useful to describe the methodologies you are familiar with, for example 'The Model for

Improvement' (https://deming.org/explore/pdsa) as a method of iterative testing. You can briefly describe projects using aim and outcomes. If you have formal fellowships or have undertaken additional training such as IHI Open School (http://www.ihi.org/education/IHIOpenSchool/pages/default.aspx) or a Quality Improvement Diploma or Masters, note the dates and qualification clearly. See Box 1.6.

Box 1.6 My Notes
- Quality Improvement training
- Quality Improvement projects
- Aims
- Outcomes

1.14   Practical Tips

The application form is a generic tool that organisations use to ensure that you meet the requirements for the role, can be short-listed and invited for an interview. Most applications describe the technical requirements necessary for the form to be accepted and may have word or character counts in text boxes. Be sure to check these before you begin and seek any clarification from the recruitment team. Less commonly organisations may use a cover letter and curriculum vitae or resume as a means of short listing. You can use the sections described in this chapter to structure your information. A well-maintained CV will make any application process easier as it provides prompts and information that will help you fill out an application form.

The application form is your opportunity to ensure that you have described your qualifications and attributes clearly and should be the foundation for your interview preparation (Table 1.4).

Give yourself plenty of time before the application deadline and be mindful of the submission timeframe, it can take a few weeks to pull together all the information and get in touch with

Table 1.4 Application checklist

• *Proofread your application*
• *Check important personal details and credentials that are requirements for shortlisting*
• *Cross-check that you have referenced essential and desirable criteria and qualifications*
• *Check the contact details for your proposed referees*
• *Ensure you have access to relevant certificates and documents*

possible referees. Online applications can be cumbersome in terms of formatting and can take longer than you anticipate especially as word count restrictions may apply to particular sections. Submission dates and times can be in 24 h clock format which can cause confusion therefore it is sensible to plan submission at least a few days before the deadline.

1.15   Well-Being

Once you get shortlisted the interview date will be confirmed. You are unlikely to perform at your best if you are tired and stressed. Exercise, eating well and taking care of yourself are part of bringing your best self not only to work every day but to an interview. Try to plan ahead so that you can get a few good nights' sleep and have had a chance to decompress from any particularly stressful work prior to your interview. This may involve looking ahead at your work rota/schedule and asking for some time off to prepare.

Visiting the Organisation and Interview Format

2

You may already be working within the organisation or applying as a new employee. Regardless of any previous experience, it is important to consider what is different about your new role. This chapter will catch you through the interview format and help you structure your preparation for a pre-interview visit.

Most organisations will offer the opportunity to have a conversation with a senior healthcare leader who you can ask about the department, the organisational commitments, goals and any areas they hope to develop in the future. This is your chance to get a feel for the organisation and a sense of how your skill set complements the existing team. It also provides insight into the organisational context, priorities, challenges and values. If you can, try and visit in person but if not a virtual visit with good preparation will also be helpful.

Preparation is important. Take time to read about the organisation: what are their corporate objectives, do they have a clear mission, culture and values statement? Most organisations will publish an annual report that will give you a flavour of their areas of delivery and in particular the areas they excel in. If you have experience that aligns with their corporate goals then the visit is an opportunity to find out more about how this might work with staff on the ground. See Box 2.1 preparing to visit an organisation pre-interview.

C. T. Lundy, *The Medical Interview Coach*,
https://doi.org/10.1007/978-3-031-16321-0_2

You may be able to get some further background on key members of the clinical department by reading their recent publications or using professional networks and social media. This can help you consider what questions you have about what it might be like to work in the department, what opportunities there are for new staff and any workplace challenges you might face. You may wish to ask if the department contributes to any national benchmarking or audit projects and if there is an expectation about the new post holder contributing to this kind of work. The department may also have a research profile in a particular field, it is useful to ask about active projects and support for research.

Box 2.1 The Coach Approach
How can you make the most of your visit?
Think about your goal… what exactly to you want to find out about the organisation, department and role?
What are the exceptions about teaching and training?
Who would you like to meet before the interview?

Most clinical areas will contribute to education and training of undergraduate students and postgraduate staff in a range of disciplines. Use your visit to ascertain what expectations there are around teaching and training.

If you have a specific area of interest you may wish to set up a meeting with a staff member who has a leadership role in that field. For example, if your interest is quality improvement you could ask to meet the organisation's quality and safety lead or if your interest is in digital health and healthcare technology you may wish to meet the chief clinical information officer. The human resources/recruitment team should be able to help you with relevant contacts for any in person or virtual visit and will be able to guide you on reimbursement for any costs incurred.

2.1   **Important Previsit Preparation**

It is important to check who you are allowed to contact in advance of the interview as you may be precluded from speaking to possible interview panel members. You may be disqualified from the process if you speak to people in the organisation in an attempt to influence the outcome of the interview in your favour, this can be referred to as 'canvassing'. The organisation will want the process to be fair to all candidates. If you are unsure about who you can speak with you can always check in advance with the recruitment team before you visit or make contact. See Boxes 2.2 and 2.3.

Box 2.2 My Notes
Key department leads
    Department commitments to service/areas for development
    Expectations of the new post holder

Box 2.3 'Coach Approach'
Some useful questions to consider asking during your visit
    How would you describe the work environment here?
    How would you describe the culture here?
    What are the service goals?
    What are you most proud of in this department?
    What do you think the working week will look like in this role?
    What types of career opportunities might I have in this organisation?
    What type of administrative support will I have in this role?
    How will my performance be measured?
    Is there support for innovation?

2.2   Practical Tips-visit Checklist

- Check with the Human Resources/Recruitment team who you are allowed to contact and what format is possible, in person or virtual.
- Have a range of dates and times in mind.
- Read relevant organisational material such as the Annual Report or other recent publications.
- Consider what questions you have about the department and team composition.
- Prepare questions about opportunities and challenges in the organisation.
- Be prepared to talk about your own relevant clinical experience and why you are interested in the role.
- Consider this the first stage of the interview. Be professional, courteous and appreciative of the staff who give you time and answer your questions.

2.3   The Interview Panel and Format

Most interviews for healthcare positions in public organisations are set up to ensure they are fair and transparent, meet employment law requirements and withstand legal scrutiny if there is a challenge to the outcome. The process will be documented, there will be a prearranged interview panel who will have undertaken appropriate training in recruitment, equality and diversity supported by a designated recruitment officer. Usually, the interview will be in a panel format which includes representatives from the clinical area of practice, a senior healthcare leader such as the lead of a department in the hospital, a senior manager and an executive director. For senior positions, the panel may include representation from an affiliated University, relevant professional body such as a Royal College in the UK, Non-Executive Director and may have a person with a non-clinical background as a Chairperson. You can check the panel format in advance.

The panel will usually have agreed to the questions and points allocated so that a fair approach can be taken to scoring candidates, a 'pass mark' is often agreed in advance. This process, including composition of the panel is usually overseen by the Human Resources/Recruitment team in most organisations to ensure all relevant standards are met in terms of fairness, equality and diversity. You will usually have a designated contact within the recruitment team. It is important that you have provided up-to-date telephone and e-mail contact details so that any information can be provided promptly. You can usually ask for information about who is likely to be on the panel and the interview format as some will include a presentation. Having advance knowledge of the panel composition provides another opportunity to prepare by identifying areas that these individuals might be focused on with respect to the advertised post.

2.4   The Virtual Interview

It may not be possible to have an in-person interview and virtual interviews are becoming much more common. It is vital to prepare for a virtual interview as if you were attending in person. You may have been using virtual platforms for clinical work, such as MS Teams or Zoom, however, you may have only used them for connection with family and friends. Do not assume that connecting with another organisation will be straightforward. Some organisations block certain platforms as part of their security process.

Recruitment and human resources professionals have had to adapt to provide healthcare panel interviews in a virtual format. It is a good idea to prepare for a virtual interview in advance to ensure that you have the best experience and reduce your stress before your interview. You should familiarise yourself with the technology that is going to be used, you can check this with the recruitment contact. Find out exactly what platform they use and ensure that your device is compatible and that you have had a few trial runs with a friend.

2.5   Virtual Interview Tips

You will be asked to confirm your identity so be prepared and have a suitable form of identification with your photograph and name clearly visible.

You can prepare for a virtual interview by ensuring your technical set up is optimised. This may involve rebooting your computer and ensuring all other programmes are closed downbefore you launch the virtual interview platform you will be using for your interview; this will stop any unwelcome alert messages from popping up and distracting you. Do this well in advance of the scheduled interview time…not 5 min beforehand as you may end up with delays as updates start to install! Turn off 'notifications and ensure all your telephones are on 'silent'. Try this in a dry run with a friend before the interview date.

Consider how you can prepare your environment. In particular, think about your background and what is going to be seen by the panel. You do not want them to be distracted by activity in the room, they should be focusing on you and your response to their questions. Lighting is important. It is not ideal to have a light source behind you as this may cast your face into shade. Think about having lamps on either side of your face or a ring light on your computer screen as this will help ensure that your face is not cast into shadow and make it easier to respond with facial cues to the panel as you listen to questions.

Another thing to think about is where to look on your home screen, check where your camera is and think about where the panel videos will appear on your device so that you have a focused place to look when responding to questions; ideally straight ahead. You can move the 'gallery' display around on your screen and it can be helpful to practice this in advance. If you require any *specific technical support* with the interview set up ensure that you have made the recruitment contact aware of this in a timely fashion. The panel may ask to see the area in front of you to ensure you do not have any notes that would give you an unfair advantage.

It is important to be prepared for glitches! We have all used technology for virtual consultations and meetings and have experienced problems, therefore at the very beginning of the interview it is useful to confirm that the panel has the correct telephone number for you and that you have a means of contacting them should the technology experience significant issues. Of course, a small pause in video can happen and you should prepare and practice so that something like this does not cause you to worry and stress during the interview. You can think in advance about what you will say to the panel when the camera reconnects, for example *'Thank you for your patience, my camera paused briefly'*.

It may be helpful to recap on the question that you are responding to, for example *'I would just like to go back to Claire's question about teamwork, I had mentioned a project I was working on that demonstrated my skills in this area....'* and continue with your response.

It is worthwhile having a notepad, pen and a glass of water to hand as sometimes in an interview we lose our train of thought because of nervousness. It is important to try and get yourself back on track, this can be a little trickier in a virtual interview as you may not see nonverbal cues just as well. If you feel that you may have gone off at a tangent, do take the opportunity to pause and ask the panel member to repeat the question so that you can ensure you are answering to the best of your ability.

A final point: give yourself the opportunity to prepare for a virtual interview in the same way you would for a face-to-face interview by providing yourself with a quiet environment where you will not be disturbed. Think about what makes you most confident in terms of your professional appearance and consider how some colours and patterns of clothing appear on the screen as some may disrupt the video quality more than others and make the screen appear a little blurry. See Table 2.1.

Consider your virtual interview set-up in well advance, ensure you know where your camera is and how you will manage your background environment. Glitches happen...but you can be prepared for them.

Table 2.1 Virtual interview checklist

• Confirm video platform to be used, ask for any support well in advance
• Install relevant IT and practice using it in advance
• Prepare your interview environment—consider your background
• Have suitable photographic identification to show the panel
• Have other information you have been asked to display, e.g. qualifications or certificates
• Consider everything you will need such as writing materials and water—try to avoid a spill!
• Provide contact details and ask for panel contact details should IT issues occur on the day of the interview

2.6   Attending an Interview in Person

Attending an interview in a new organisation can cause anxiety so take time to ensure that you know where the venue is and that you have given yourself sufficient time to get there. Ensure you do not have significant work prior to the interview that may result in you arriving late or being emotional or upset in any way that could adversely affect your performance.

It is generally expected that you would dress in an appropriate manner for the role on a day-to-day basis—most organisations provide guidance on expected dress code for the work environment, it is worth reviewing this information prior to attendance. Most candidates will adopt a more formal approach to dress for an interview. Consider what will look professional and still be comfortable!

Ensure that you have copies of any required information such as identification papers, passport and professional qualifications.

2.7   Unseen Presentations

Interviews may include 'unseen' presentation topics. This provides the panel with an opportunity to see you respond to a challenge and develop a coherent discussion around a topic. It is worth practicing this before the interview and you will usually be provided with advance warning that this may take place and the materials you will have at your disposal to prepare, e.g. a notepad, whiteboard or electronic device. You may be able to get information on the topic area to allow some specific preparation. Some tips for developing a presentation include:

- Focus on the question you have been asked and the time you have to prepare.
- Who is the audience—are you providing information for a mixed medical and non-medical panel.
- What information do you want to convey—present coherent short points that you can elaborate on as required.
- Highlight personal knowledge, skills and training in the topic area
- Describe the relevance for patient care and the organisation.
- Summarise and ask for questions.

2.8   Other Practical Tips...

2.8.1   Introductions

The panel will greet you and introduce themselves usually mentioning briefly where they work and their role in the organisation.

2.8.2   Answering Questions: Getting Your Message Across

Ideally, you should have a structure to your answers. Whilst you will be able to prepare for some questions in a detailed way, there will be some nuances to how they are asked. It is critical to listen carefully and you can ask for the question to be repeated so you are sure you have grasped the important areas. Take a moment to think how to respond. This pause is an important chance for you to formulate a structure for your answer. Practice will make this much easier!

It is vital to remember that you must respect patient confidentiality and the reputation of professional colleagues and organisations when you are preparing any answers that involve clinical scenarios.

2.8.3   Answering Questions

Most of us remember things in three's. Aim to deliver a clear response in approximately three main areas. One suggested way of delivering your answer in this way is to outline at the beginning what you are going to say so that the panel has a clear idea of your thought process, provide detail in the body of your answer and then summarise what you have said in a couple of lines. You can then ask if the panel would like you to clarify any of your responses or if they have any further questions, for example ' would you like me to clarify any particular areas of my answer?', or 'I would be happy to expand on this topic further if you have any further questions?'

An example of a response to a question on your involvement in benchmarking or audit:

'Thank you, I have been involved in two national audits and a number of local audits during my training. I would like to share my experience of how audit contributes to quality and safety and how I have participated in audit projects that made a real difference to patient care…

Provide further detail on one or two projects describing the purpose of the work, the team involved, your role, stakeholder engagement, outcomes and what this led to in terms of safety and quality of care…

In summary, I hope I have explained the very positive experience I have had in working with the wider team assessing our departmental outcomes in relation to national standards. This work led to better team understanding of the expected standards of care and further investment in the service.'

This style of answer is clear and easy to follow, the messages are obvious and allow the interviewer to note and score your responses in relation to key areas.

2.8.4   Story Telling

Other styles include a 'story telling' approach. This can be particularly powerful if you are trying to convey a sense of your leadership style, your approach to challenging situations and your ability to collaborate with others. When considering a clinical scenario or challenge that can lend itself to this engaging style of answer consider the following tips to help you structure your response. This style requires well-thought-out scenarios that you are comfortable to share, try to avoid very emotional examples that may impact on your ability to stay calm.

There are a number of narrative approaches but a familiar one that will engage the listener is often described as 'The Hero's Journey'.

- The location/context—take the audience on the journey with you…
- The call to action
- Mentorship
- Allies
- The challenge
- Overcoming the challenge
- Rewards/benefits
- Demonstration of learning/new found wisdom

The Socratic approach to posing sub-questions that you then answer can also be an interesting style of narrative. For example… 'during my training I focused on learning a particular surgical technique, why was this so important to me? I knew that it was recognised as providing patients with better outcomes such as reduced post operative pain and quicker discharge time'.

As you work through this book the 'coach approach' sections will help you develop a deeper understanding of the knowledge you have in each area of practice. As you start to practice your answers you will start to identify which narrative style feels most comfortable and natural for you.

2.8.5 The Opening Question…Why Are You the Best Person for This Job?

Most healthcare interviews start with an opening question that allows the candidate to share their clinical background and also settle into the interview. It is usually asked by a representative from a professional organisation such as a University or Royal College in the UK. It can be asked in a variety of ways such as:

- Can you take us through the areas of your CV that are relevant to this role?
- Can you tell us how you fulfil the criteria for this role?
- Please explain how your training is relevant for this position.

This is your opportunity to showcase your training and experience and describe how you are the best fit for the role. It is useful to really think about this question in advance as it is predictable and you can score well on it with thoughtful preparation which highlights your unique experience, skills and competencies.

Think about the key areas of clinical skill that are set out as essential criteria for the role and highlight these in a coherent way that tells a short story of your knowledge and skill acquisition in the last few years. A narrative approach is more interesting for the listener than a recitation of your qualifications.

You may wish to consider packaging your training journey into the main areas of practice to make it interesting for the panel and clear in demonstrating that you have all the relevant skills.

For example, Thank you for the opportunity to share my experience, I would like to summarise my relevant academic and clinical qualifications and my main areas of interest that are closely aligned to this role.

I was awarded my Medical Degree from Queens University and a Master's Degree from Sheffield Hallam University in addition I have completed training in Clinical Leadership, Quality Improvement and Coaching.

I started my paediatric training in 2000. I quickly progressed into a specialist neurology training post in London following completion of basic training and my membership exams. During specialist training i develped an interest in children wiht neurodisability and completed further qualifications in this field. I undertook research and have published papers in peer-reviewed journals and presented the work nationally and internationally….

On a personal level, my values align with the organisation. I have demonstrated my commitment to improving patient care through research and innovation and I have supported and led clinical teams in the delivery of a shared vision of high-quality care which has achieved national recognition. My style of teamwork and leadership is to be curious about how to improve and to collaborate with all colleagues inspired by this shared purpose. I believe a compassionate approach to both patients and staff results in the best care and working environment.

I hope that I have demonstrated that I have both the clinical expertise and knowledge to support the department in delivering excellent care for children with neurological conditions. I will bring additional skills in service development and innovation and an enthusiastic approach to working within the existing team.

2.8.6   Interview Practice

The more you prepare and practice, the more comfortable and relaxed you will feel during an interview. In the months before the interview identify opportunities to present at team meetings and meet with senior colleagues to discuss your work within the team and your possible new role. Each of these meetings or presentations should be seen as a 'mini-interview' as you can use them to think about how you might present to a panel and also some of the important areas that may come up as questions. Familiarising yourself with presenting in a formal way will help you if your interview includes a presentation and will build your confidence.

Practice with an interview coach or trusted colleague can be very beneficial. This provides an invaluable opportunity to articulate your answers and move away from written preparation and reading around topics. Ask for feedback and using this constructive criticism look for further learning or coaching support.

Learning answers can sound very rehearsed and unnatural: focus on being able to flex your examples and experience in a more conversational, authentic style. A very rehearsed answer may not address key points in the question and you are likely to score poorly. Do not be afraid to pause and ask if the question can be repeated so that you have time to think and consider how best to answer. Saying your answers out loud and recording them using platforms such as MSTeams or Zoom is another helpful tool in preparing for an interview and will allow you to review how coherent you are and if you have clearly demonstrated your knowledge and skills or omitted to talk about key areas of expertise. See reflective feedback template Box 2.4.

Box 2.4 Reflective Feedback Template
- Did I answer the question by demonstrating an understanding of the topic area? If relevant referencing local/national guidance.
- Did I highlight my relevant skills that meet the essential/desirable criteria in this area?
- Was there an example that described my personal approach? Comment on the use of language demonstrating values, behaviours and leadership and communication style.
- Was there a description of any additional qualifications/skills relevant to the area?
- Did I highlight personal/team learning/innovation if relevant?
- Did I summarise?

Clinical Skills at Interview 3

The most important part of any healthcare interview is when the panel tries to get a sense of your ability to fulfil the requirements of the post and your style of healthcare delivery. As you use the coach approach in this chapter you will develop a better understanding of how to present your skillset using a powerful, coherent and narrative style. The clinical section of your interview is 'competency' based and it is important that your examples provide a clear outline of your ability. There are ways to structure competency-focussed examples, one approach is to use *STARR-*.

Situation—the context of your example, e.g. where you were working and the team
Task—what did you need to do?
Action—what clinical skills you used and how you delivered the care/intervention?
Result—what was the outcome for the patient/team?
Review—what did you learn?

C. T. Lundy, *The Medical Interview Coach*,
https://doi.org/10.1007/978-3-031-16321-0_3

3.1   Your Clinical Skills

When working as a healthcare professional, personal values such as openness and honesty, compassion and commitment to excellence often align with the healthcare 'organisational values'. The behaviours we exhibit in the workplace demonstrate our values in a practical way day to day; kindness, compassion, listening to others and good team work skills. Patient safety is paramount and patient care is better when there is good communication and teamwork underpinned by compassion and a commitment to delivering the highest quality of care. Many healthcare organisations are now incorporating questions or assessments that allow a panel to identify if the candidate's values are aligned to that of the organisation. This approach aims to identify individuals who will work towards shared goals in a team and help deliver the safest and most effective care. When preparing for an interview it is useful to read the organisation's statements on 'mission' and 'values'.

When thinking about your clinical skills, it is important to frame your answers around your personal style of healthcare delivery for each area; consider how you can demonstrate that you are safety focussed as well as curious about how to improve care, patient centred and a team player. Good healthcare requires a doctor to be able to work not only in partnership with patients and clients but with the wider team. The General Medical Council UK clearly outlines this in the guidance on Duties of a Doctor (https://www.gmc-uk.org/ethical-guidance/ethical-guidance-for-doctors/good-medical-practice/duties-of-a-doctor) A consultation is in progress in the UK with an expected update in 2023 which may have a further emphasis on leadership and partnership working with patients and more focus on identifying what matters to patients. There are similar themes in healthcare regulators worldwide, you should familiarise yourself with the relevant terminology particularly if you are moving country and reflect on the most current guidance.

Healthcare has changed rapidly in terms of mode of delivery in the last number of years particularly following the COVID-19 pandemic. At times owing to resources, restrictions or staffing constraints we have not always been able to deliver care in the way in which we have trained or in the way in which we would most like to. However, demonstrating your ability to adapt and respond to the changing needs of the population is an important clinical skill. Consider examples where you can describe the flexible and adaptable approach that you have taken in delivering high-quality patient care and overcome challenges in your environment. See Box 3.1 Try using the 'STARR' competency-based approach to structure your examples. See Table 3.1.

When we consider the values described in healthcare organisations around the world and specifically within the UK, most

---

Box 3.1 'Coach Approach'
- What was the organisational/clinical setting?
- What clinical care needs were you trying to address?
- What action did you take?
- Why was this important?
- Who was able to assist you with any service/treatment model changes?
- How did you assess the benefits for patients and measure any adverse outcomes?
- Were there personal attributes that helped you work well within your team to deliver the desired change?
- Can you identify how your personal approach links with organisational values?
- Did this work align with organisational healthcare priorities?
- What did you learn?

---

organisations will be looking for individuals who can demonstrate a commitment to compassionate care, an open and honest approach, an ability to work well in a team, in partnership with patients and deliver excellence. When you are looking at the

Table 3.1 Situation—The context of your example, e.g. where you were working and the team

Task—what did you need to do?
Action—what clinical skills you used and how you delivered the care/intervention?
Result—what was the outcome for the patient/team?
Review—what did you learn?

corporate information for any organisation identify their corporate values and consider how well they are aligned to your own. It is likely that values-based interview questions will become more prevalent in the years ahead as there is an increasing recognition that the ability to work well within a team and behave in a manner aligned to the desired organisational culture results in better outcomes for patient care and happier teams.

3.2   Demonstrating Your Values in Clinical Practice

'Compassionate care' is something that sounds good but what does it really mean? Compassion is an ability to recognise the suffering of others and as healthcare professionals, we need to do more than just recognise, we need to move to alleviate that suffering. Demonstrating compassionate care means that you have to clearly describe your ability to listen to your patients and understand from their perspective what they really need to manage their condition, understand the treatment options and potential outcomes.

Workplace compassion is equally important. How can you demonstrate an ability to behave with compassion within a team environment? Do you help other members of the team deliver care? Are you aware of the contribution of other team members? Do you recognise when a colleague is under pressure and try to provide support or signpost them to appropriate resources? Being able to describe situations like this in relation to clinical work will give the panel a sense of how you use your emotional intelligence.

Working well together means working well within a team, with patients, clients and their families. In practice, we need to consider how our clinical work is best delivered as part of the wider team. In your preparation think of examples that will allow you to demonstrate how you deliver effective care. Describe your ability to work well within the healthcare team considering both your immediate clinical team and colleagues within the wider healthcare system such as other departments, managerial colleagues and commissioning colleagues such as those in government roles which impact on population health. See Box 3.2.

Box 3.2 'Coach Approach

Consider examples where you have demonstrated your values. For example, think about a time when you recognised the need for a compassionate approach to a challenging situation, or when you developed a project to support the delivery of a better standard of care.

How do you ensure the contributions of patients and colleagues in clinical decision-making?

Why is this important to you and the organisation?

Is there a leader or mentor you admire in terms of their style of leadership/healthcare provision? Think about what you observe and how that makes you feel.

Have you undertaken any leadership development during your training? How did that help you?

Did you do things differently or amplify certain behaviours?

How would others describe your style of clinical leadership?

3.3 Patient Engagement, Openness and Transparency

Consider ways in which you can demonstrate your ability to work well with patients/clients to deliver services in a way that is most effective, accessible and fit for purpose in the twenty-first century. Some organisations will reference terms such as co-production and patient engagement in their corporate literature. These are umbrella terms describing how patients as service users had direct input into a project or service development. Patient engagement can take a number of forms such as focus groups, daily feedback on a ward or outpatient unit, patient advisors and user groups. You should expect clinical service questions to draw on these themes.

In line with regulatory guidance, organisations and clinical units such as primary care providers will have corporate documentation highlighting their emphasis and duties around openness, honesty and transparency. It is essential that you are able to demonstrate your ability to communicate with openness and honesty when dealing with a clinical situation. It is also important to think of examples where openness and honesty have played a part in learning from any errors or situations when clinical care did not go as you or your team had hoped. Consider your learning style in relation to this type of issue, being able to demonstrate a 'growth mindset' is more likely to lead to a deeper understanding of the problem and have a higher chance of developing solutions that will deliver improvements in care.

3.4 Delivering High-Quality Clinical Care

Many organisations will describe high quality or excellence in healthcare as a core value. Healthcare professionals are also ambitious for the care they deliver to patients. The questions around safe clinical care allow you the opportunity to showcase work that you have undertaken which describes your commitment to delivering the best possible care to the patients that you serve. Using the competency focussed approach think about examples that allow you to explain this in terms of assessment of patient outcomes and celebration of success with your team or the wider organisation.

3.4.1   Reflective Exercise: Growth Mindset Versus Fixed Mindset

This exercise will help you formulate a structured approach to describing learning from different challenging or adverse situations.

Consider a situation where you have had to respond to a workplace challenge or critical feedback from a colleague or serice user. Go through the statements below and see if your approach to the situation demonstrated a growth mindset or were you or others in the team demonstrating more of a fixed mindset.

3.4.2   Growth Mindset

I enjoyed considering new ways of working.
I found this an opportunity to grow on a personal level.
I learnt from this experience.
The feedback was helpful.
I found the challenge inspired me to improve.

3.4.3   Fixed Mindset

I do not really like being challenged.
I found the situation so frustrating I gave up.
The feedback felt threatening.
I cannot do this.
I find it is better to stick to my area of expertise.
This feedback is not relevant.

Consider examples when you have felt really proud about the care you and your team have delivered—what was good about it in terms of results for the patient and outcomes for the team—e.g. did the team build a stronger relationship through training and education and working towards a shared goal? Think about how this might influence your future delivery of healthcare. Using the template below as a coaching guide, work through clinical situations that you would be happy to talk about during an interview that will help you showcase your unique skillset. See Box 3.3.

Box 3.3 Coach Approach
- Outline the clinical/organisational scenario.
- What was your clinical contribution/action? What was important about the clinical care in terms of your skillset? Align this to the essential and desirable clinical criteria.
- How did you know the outcome was good? Were you able to define the desired standard of care and benchmark it against a national standard?
- How did the patient feel? What feedback did you obtain?
- Did that influence practice?
- Developing your personal contribution: how can you describe this in terms of your professional skills and competencies and any further learning or support you can bring to the department/organisation?
- What do you feel helped overall in terms of the values and behaviour of the team?
- Do you feel you showed leadership?
- Can you describe how your style of leadership and actions contributed to the successful outcome?
- Was your team recognised by colleagues or the organisation? How did you celebrate success?
- Has this work lead on to service changes that are now embedded in practice?
- How have you applied this experience to other areas of your work?

3.4.4   Example Answer Suggested Structure: Identify the Key Actions You Took and the Team Approach

This is not intended to be a detailed model answer however it will provide a suggested structure for describing your approach to addressing an important issue?

In my area of practice with children with complex neurological disability there was a clear need for a more cohesive approach to practice that brought the patient and family goals into alignment with service providers in community and local paediatric consultants. We were also aware that care was at times disjointed and we needed to work in line with NICE guidance for young people with cerebral palsy.

How Did We Approach the Challenge?

Working as a team we benchmarked against gold standard services elsewhere including the UK and internationally. We piloted a new interdisciplinary model where children and families identified goals and we provided specialist assessment and targeted treatment ideas…I brought new medical skills to the team which opened up a new opportunity for service provision.

What Were the Financial and Personnel Considerations?

I worked closely with managerial and commissioning colleagues to share the vision for holistic assessment in line with national benchmarks. …The team measured goal-focussed outcomes so that we could report any improvements clearly… The team was excited by the opportunity to work towards better engagement with this population, they enjoyed the chance to learn together and acquire new skills. We were able to describe improved outcomes in a range of areas such as patient satisfaction, pain management and improving functional ability.

Were There Training Needs?

During the early phase of this work, I reached out to expert colleagues based in other centres for guidance and support. This enabled our team to collaborate with national centres of excellence and deliver training and support to local colleagues to build skills and confidence…The generosity of highly skilled colleagues who willingly helped with additional training helped our training groups blossom into a regional learning network. We succeeded in making the case for permanent funding from healthcare commissioners and have received recognition locally and nationally for our work…

What Did Families and Professionals Think of the Work?
Families were delighted to share their practical goals and were pleased when they saw how activities of daily living could become easier for their children. Children liked that there were fewer appointments in the hospital.

Professionals felt that they had a more focussed approach to this cohort of patients and were pleased that through the development of new skills and better collaborative working they were able to see improvements in patient care. They felt empowered and community providers are now active contributors to teaching and training in our regional learning network.

How Did the Work Align with Local and National Healthcare Priorities?
The work was identified as supporting organisational and regional goals for early intervention and linked to National Guidelines for management of Cerebral Palsy in the UK. The team's success was also due to the clear vision for improving outcomes through a collaborative interdisciplinary approach to treatment. Extended team members in local child development clinics embraced the vision and worked towards the well-described outcomes…This affiliative style of leadership has led to this model of practice becoming the standard for our region and the learning network continues to flourish and grow.

3.5   Using Examples

The coach approach will assist you in developing examples as you work through each chapter. Spending time now considering times or places where you learnt a lot can help you think 'on the spot' in the interview!

If you get stuck try and keep a few key words in mind:

Why?
Who?
How?
Results?
Learning?

3.6   In Summary

Clinical skills questions afford you the best opportunity to share your unique abilities. Remember to approach these questions thoughtfully. Your message should be easily understood by both the lay members of the panel as well as the clinical specialists. Keep your responses structured with clear information that describes your clinical skillset and provides insight into your personal approach to healthcare.

3.7   Clinical Skills/Competencies Checklist

- Look at the essential and desirable criteria—map to your clinical skills and competencies.

- Research the corporate values—do these align with your values and how will you describe this?
- What examples do you have where you demonstrated competence and confidence in the essential and desirable clinical skills?
- Consider how you will describe your style of healthcare delivery in relation to these examples.
- How can you demonstrate your commitment to high-quality care using these examples?

Sample Questions Chapter 3

- Tell us how you will assist in the delivery of improved patient care in the next 5 years?
- Using examples describe what you can bring to the team in terms of clinical expertise and how will this benefit patients and colleagues?
- How would you describe your approach to the delivery of high-quality care in your field of expertise?
- What do you feel are the biggest challenges ahead in this clinical field and how will you be able to help this organisation address them?
- What is your experience in developing and delivering new models of care delivery?
- Can you tell us why your clinical skills are relevant to this position?
- Can you tell us how your clinical skills will help improve patient care in our unit?

Leading Healthcare Teams 4

A new opportunity to lead a healthcare team as a medical consultant or in a new clinical leadership role is an exciting chance to amplify your clinical impact. The coach approach in this chapter will help you to develop compelling narratives about your personal leadership journey, your style of leadership and your ability to lead a team in complex systems.

4.1 Background Knowledge

Clinical leadership has been brought into focus in recent years as a key component of the ability of an organisation to deliver high-quality care. Sadly, when clinicians are not in a position to lead, patients can experience adverse outcomes such as those described in the Mid Staffordshire report in the UK (https://www.medical-council.ie/news-and-publications/reports/guide-to-professional-conduct-and-ethics-for-registered-medical-practitioners-amended-.pdf; https://www.gov.uk/government/publications/report-of-the-mid-staffordshire-nhs-foundation-trust-public-inquiry). There are additional recognised negative impacts for teams working in 'toxic' environments with poor staff morale, poor outcomes and reduced well-being.

The GMC report 2019 'Caring for doctors, caring for patients' authored by Mike West and Denise Coia (https://www.medical-

C. T. Lundy, *The Medical Interview Coach*,
https://doi.org/10.1007/978-3-031-16321-0_4

board.gov.au/codes-guidelines-policies/code-of-conduct.aspx) describes the importance of doctor's well-being in three main areas, 'Autonomy, Belonging and Competence'. A key part of 'belonging' is organisational culture and leadership; the report highlights the need for all healthcare organisations in the UK to look at mechanisms that 'ensure clinical leads and other leaders of doctors at all levels in the healthcare system are recruited, selected, developed, assessed and supported to model compassionate and collective leadership'. Other regulators have similar frameworks, for example the Irish Medical Council focusses on 'Professionalism' and highlights a doctor's duty to ensure they work well with patients and colleagues, demonstrate good communication and advocate for the needs of patients in a culture of safety. The Australian Medical Council describes the importance of self-reflection and self-awareness as a part of professionalism and provides clear guidance on the expectations of the public regarding doctor's behaviours with respect to their work.

https://www.medicalcouncil.ie/news-and-publications/reports/guide-to-professional-conduct-and-ethics-for-registered-medical-practitioners-amended-.pdf (https://www.gmc-uk.org/ethical-guidance/ethical-guidance-for-doctors/leadership-and-management-for-all-doctors).

https://www.medicalboard.gov.au/codes-guidelines-policies/code-of-conduct.aspx (https://www.gov.uk/government/publications/the-7-principles-of-public-life/the-7-principles-of-public-life%2D%2D2).

This suggests that recruitment processes will have an increased focus on a candidate's ability to demonstrate both interest and capability in developing their personal leadership skills. You can read a number of reports that provide useful guidance on the clinical leadership skills expected from medical practitioners including the GMC guidance on Leadership and Management for all Doctors (2012) (https://www.gmc-uk.org/-/media/documents/caring-for-doctors-caring-for-patients_pdf-80706341.pdf). The Seven Principles of Public Life (https://www.gov.uk/government/publications/the-7-principles-of-public-life/the-7-principles-of-public-life%2D%2D2) outlines the expected behaviour of those in public roles in the UK: selflessness, integrity, openness, accountability, honesty and leadership. Literature developed by the organisation 'Faculty of Medical Leadership in Medicine' FMLM, in the UK outlines a framework of leadership behaviour in the document 'Leadership and Management Standards for Medical Professionals'. Dr. Peter Lees from FMLM has described the increasing awareness of 'the increased accountability and responsibility that doctors have with respect to the effectiveness and efficiency of healthcare delivery, advice, safety and quality'. The GMC document Duties of a Doctor (latest update 2019) (https://www.gmc-uk.org/ethical-guidance/ethical-guidance-for-doctors/good-medical-practice/duties-of-a-doctor) also emphasises the importance of good team work and collaboration with patients and colleagues. A consultation is currently in progress with an expected update in 2023 which may have a further emphasis on leadership skills for doctors and partnership working with patients.

When reading these documents reflect on your personal leadership experience in recent years. Use the following questions as a

Box 4.1 Coach Approach
Using an example describe how you have demonstrated the professional values and leadership behaviours expected in healthcare?

- Outline your understanding of the healthcare values/behaviours and reference national guidance such as GMC.
- Develop a workplace example to provide context, describe a challenging team-based scenario, outline the leadership approach you took and how your behaviour in that setting made a difference.
- Can you describe the impact on patient care and your team?
- Was your approach aligned with the national/organisational values/behaviours you mentioned in your opening statement?
- Using an example describe your clinical leadership style?

template to structure your response to a question on clinical leadership. See Box 4.1.

4.1.1 Your Leadership Style

Provide a short overview of your understanding of the various clinical leadership styles and how clinicians often have to flex and adapt depending on the clinical context. When considering your answer consider the following reflective prompts:

- When have you observed good clinical leadership? How did it make you and others feel?
- How would you describe your clinical leadership style?
- How would others describe your clinical leadership style?
- Can leadership style impact on team outcomes? Think of examples.
- How does lack of leadership impact on patient care?
- How does poor leadership affect a team?
- How can you demonstrate self-awareness? Think of times when you demonstrated a willingness to learn/improve.

4.2 Leadership Style: What the Research Tells Us?

Leadership style is an important area to consider in your preparation. This section highlights some key recommended reading in the field. If you have had the opportunity to undertake leadership development training you will recognise that this is an expanding area of knowledge and the healthcare-related leadership literature is evolving.

In his sentinel paper in the Harvard Business Review, Daniel Goleman [1] comments on a variety of leadership styles: *Directive, Visionary, Affiliative, Participative, Pace Setting and Coaching.* 'Pace setting' is noted to be more common in healthcare professionals and Goleman and colleagues describe the ability of the most effective leaders to use different styles dependent on context. The best leaders exhibit visionary, participative and collaborative behaviours that enable and empower their teams. Leadership theory continues to evolve and the impact of personality has been described in work undertaken by Judge et al. [2]. Their work describes openness to experience, extroversion, neuroticism, agreeableness and conscientiousness and their impact on behaviour when under pressure and the effect this may have on others. There is some correlation to the Myers–Briggs analysis that has been used fairly widely. If you have not had the opportunity to undertake an assessment like this it may be worth considering a 360 evaluation so you can reflect on your strengths and the areas that you would like to develop as part of your personal learning. The NHS provides a free 360 assessment if you register on their Leadership Academy site. There are other companies that offer feedback tools and your organisation may also offer feedback tools as part of annual appraisal processes. Additional links are provided at the end of this chapter for NHS leadership resources.

The *NHS healthcare leadership model* breaks expectations down into actions that demonstrate benefits for patients and teams and provides a useful reflective template as you consider times in your career when you have demonstrated leadership capability and behaviours for example:

- *Inspiring shared purpose*
- *Leading with care*
- *Evaluating information*
- *Connecting the service*
- *Sharing the vision*
- *Engaging the team*
- *Holding to account*
- *Developing capability*
- *Influencing for results*

You can use the leadership model as a template to consider examples of times when you have demonstrated leadership in key areas.

https://www.leadershipacademy.nhs.uk/wp-content/uploads/2014/10/NHSLeadership-LeadershipModel-colour.pdf

As Daniel Goleman said… *leadership is like golf, it's one game but you have to choose the right club at the right moment for the next shot.* Your interview is an opportunity to share your leadership style and the approach you have taken in various settings.

Chapter 4 Sample Questions Healthcare Leadership

- Tell us about your clinical leadership style and how it impacts on patient care?
- Using examples describe your approach to leading a clinical team.
- How have you approached a conflict situation within a clinical team?
- What leadership behaviours do you think are most important in healthcare and why?
- Using an example describe how you have shown leadership in relation to clinical care.
- Using examples can you describe why compassion is important in healthcare?
- How do you demonstrate collaborative and compassionate leadership in your day-to-day practice?
- Tell us about your approach to leading a change in patient care delivery?

References

1. 'Leadership that gets results'. Daniel Goleman. Harvard Business Review March–April 2000.
2. Judge TA, et al. Personality and leadership: a qualitative and quantitative review. J Appl Psychol. 2002;87(4):765–80. https://doi.org/10.1037//0021-9010.87.4.765. Copyright 2002 by the American Psychological Association, Inc. 0021-9010/02/$5.00

Additional Leadership Resources

https://www.leadershipacademy.nhs.uk
https://www.gov.uk/government/publications/health-and-social-care-review-leadership-for-a-collaborative-and-inclusive-future/leadership-for-a-collaborative-and-inclusive-future
https://www.leadershipacademy.nhs.uk/our-leadership-way-html/
https://www.england.nhs.uk/wp-content/uploads/2020/07/We-Are-The-NHS-Action-For-All-Of-Us-FINAL-March-21.pdf

Team Work in Healthcare 5

The last chapter helped you to develop your ideas and examples around good leadership in healthcare. As a medical leader, you also need the ability to help your team deliver on shared organisational and national healthcare strategies. In practice, this requires clinicians to demonstrate excellent teamwork skills as well as leadership skills. Using the coach approach in this chapter you will focus on describing your personal approach to teamwork, why it is important and the difference good teamwork can make in delivering patient care.

5.1 Background Knowledge

In everyday work healthcare professionals need to be able to both lead a team and work within a team. Increasingly the concept of 'team' in healthcare is becoming blurred as specialty teams interface with so many other teams within an organisation and in the wider community setting. The GMC concepts of 'Everyday leadership' 2019 described by Vance, Burford and Kehoe (https://www.gmc-uk. org/-/media/documents/everyday-leadership-12_12_19_pdf-83469618.pdf) from Newcastle University note the changing medical environment which has been influenced by complexity, technology, governance arrangements and workforce challenges. They suggest that healthcare organisations should focus on a *collective leader-*

C. T. Lundy, *The Medical Interview Coach*,
https://doi.org/10.1007/978-3-031-16321-0_5

ship' approach where all team members have a shared responsibility for organisational goals and a focus on continual learning and patient care alongside high levels of communication which allow teams to achieve shared understanding and solve problems. There is recognition that individuals will need support in terms of opportunities to develop the skills to lead a team effectively and on a practical level that there is sufficient time allocated to fulfil the commitments of the role. The NHS leadership framework highlighted in Chap. 3 reflects this collective leadership approach. There is increasing evidence around the importance of developing better self-awareness and emotional intelligence in order to lead teams well.

There has been a huge amount of research into what makes a healthcare team effective and safe. You can be certain that there will be a number of questions in your interview that present opportunities to describe your teamwork skills and approach to leading a team. It is worth spending some time thinking about your experience of working within a team that you felt demonstrated a good model of teamwork and equally considering times when you felt you may have been working within a 'pseudo team'.

In their research West and Lyupovniko describe the different aspects of a fully functional team and note that 'real teams' work closely together in a tightly coordinated way, demonstrating interdependence, have shared objectives which are clear and agreed by the team and meet regularly to systemically review their performance and adapt future team objectives and care processes accordingly- demonstrating reflexivity.

'Pseudo teams' in contrast consist of members who work largely on their own. There is little requirement to interact or communicate with each other. The objectives which healthcare team members report their team are working towards are largely disparate and healthcare team members rarely meet together to exchange information and reflect on performance. All of this leads to little or no innovation in care processes.

West further comments that members of pseudo teams report witnessing higher levels of error, incidents and near misses, more harassment, bullying and abuse from staff and patients and report lower levels of well-being and higher stress than members of real teams. In contrast, research suggests that real team characteristics result in improvements in healthcare and better patient safety.

It is worth considering the types of teams within which you have worked. During medical training doctors will have worked within teams that are perhaps more unidisciplinary. However, when moving to a consultant role, primary care or a new leadership role you may find that there is more diversity of staff from different professional backgrounds and an expectation of collaborative interdisciplinary working.

Hollenbeck et al. 2012 [2] describe the different extent to which all team members are involved in the team decision-making process. Some teams have come together over a long period of time and appear to be very stable. Hollenbeck also reports that other teams may be formed as a 'one-shot team' to deliver something new. It is recognised that the teams who work together regularly over a long period may have the opportunity to develop more effective team processes which impact positively on quality and safety of patient care. Teams that are focused on a shared purpose typically report less issues with staff well-being and conflict and are more likely to deliver an organisational goals. See Box 5.1.

Reflect on your personal experience of different decision-making styles in your current team and in previous posts:

- *What did you observe/feel was the most effective decision-making approach in particular situations?*
- *Can you relate this to leadership style, values and behaviours of individuals in the team?*

Box 5.1 'Coach Approach'

- What did you notice about the processes in place for communication within, for example an on-call team?
- Did you use a standardised safety brief or handover tool to assist with planning and sharing information?
- If you worked regularly in an outpatient service team, you may have experience of a regular weekly planning meeting and a governance meeting to share learning.

> - Consider what structured communication provides in the team context.
> - Why is it important for patient care and what have you contributed to this area?

Consider what types of teams you have worked in. For example, during your out of hours or 'on-call' you may have worked within a 'One-Shot team' to deal with an emergency or perhaps during the pandemic you were part of a new team that worked together for a short period. You may have had an opportunity to work in a stable multidisciplinary team.

What did you notice about the ways in which the different types of team operated in terms of decision-making?

5.2   Multidisciplinary Team Working

During your training or in permanent employment you may have had more opportunities to work within multidisciplinary or inter-disciplinary team environment for 6 months or more. Can you describe the team's purpose and goals? Did the team have alignment with organisational purpose and regional priorities and goals? Think about this in the context of the GMC document duties of a doctor and the focus on collaborative working.

5.3   Team Vision and Goal Setting

In your role as a team lead, you may have communicated the vision for that team and worked together to develop a shared agreement around the work that the team will then do. Achieving a vision for better care and patient outcomes over time usually involves the development of clear team goals that form the steps in the team journey. The GMC provides useful guidance for team-work, behaviour and ethical principles (https://www.gmc-uk.org/ethical-guidance/ethical-guidance-for-doctors/good-medical-practice/duties-of-a-doctor;   https://www.gmc-uk.org/ethical-

guidance/ethical-guidance-for-doctors/good-medical-practice).
See Box 5.2.

Box 5.2 'Coach Approach"
Reflect on a time when you have either been involved in
sharing a vision for a team such as working on a new project
or delivering services in a new way.

How did you build the will for change?

How did you decide what goals and outcomes would be
measured to demonstrate success?

What challenges did you and the team have to overcome?

Research from organisational development companies such as
Zenger Folkman (https://zengerfolkman.com) provide some guidance on the most effective way to set team goals. If these are
mapped out in a Venn diagram the area in the centre demonstrates
the areas of overlap in all three areas which are where team is
most likely to be successful in achieving organisational goals
whilst also enjoying their work.

1. Organisational needs—client needs and organisational standards.
2. Competence—skills and attributes of the team members.
3. Passion—areas the team enjoys.

Try mapping out these areas with your team and organisation
in mind.

As highlighted in Chap. 3 on leadership, Goleman suggests the
most effective leaders demonstrate participative and collaborative
styles of working, drawing on the inputs, experience and knowledge of both the immediate team members and subject matter
experts within their organisation and beyond. They are able to
encourage and empower team members to deliver on shared goals
within agreed timeframes. Where the team appears to be going off
track a 'real' team environment will have structures and processes
in place that allow time for the team to check in and adjust a strategy or delivery processes if required.

If some team members are struggling to achieve their goals within the service or project other team members may need to consider how they can help. They will need to understand why that person is unable to achieve their agreed role. This may require a compassionate approach as team members may be experiencing difficulty for any number of reasons including personal concerns, issues with confidence, lack of communication around team goals or unrealistic timeframes.

When you are preparing how to describe your style of team-working, it may be useful to break this down into a memorable message. The teamwork guru Patrick Lencioni from the Table Group (https://www.tablegroup.com) has a catchy description for the ideal team player: *'humble, hungry, smart'*. We can break this down into a description of behaviour: humility is the ability to ask for help when we have reached our own personal limitations; the ideal team player will work within their capability and demonstrate their competence to do the work extremely well but will also have the awareness to ask for help to ensure the team achieve the agreed goal. Working within a real team with good psychological safety enables this kind of behaviour.

Lencioni also highlights the importance of team players who are 'hungry'. These individuals share an enthusiasm and interest in delivering the work and show enjoyment when working within a team environment. They are keen to learn and support others. When considering the most successful team member, competency and the willingness to continue to learn are extremely important, particularly within the healthcare environment. Lencioni recognises that we often continue to learn within the work environment and the ideal team player has the capacity and capability to continue to develop new skills.

5.4   Psychological Safety in Healthcare Teams

Delivering the highest standards of care requires teams to work well together, sometimes which involves challenging models of working or behaviour in the workplace. You will recognise that in order to do this a workplace needs to feel 'psychologically safe' otherwise employees will be afraid to speak up. Amy Edmondson has carried out significant research in this area and the Institute for Healthcare Improvement has developed resources to help healthcare professionals understand more about psychological safety in the workplace and how it can impact on care delivery and patient safety. See Box 5.3 (http://www.ihi.org/education/IHIOpenSchool/resources/Pages/AudioandVideo/Amy-Edmondson-Three-Ways-to-Create-Psychological-Safety-in-Health-Care.aspx;   http://www.ihi.org/resources/Pages/IHIWhitePapers/Framework-Safe-Reliable-Effective-Care.aspx).

Box 5.3 'Coach Approach'

Using the concepts of clinical competence, teamwork skills and leadership consider your experience of working within a team that you felt was a real team. Were you able to demonstrate these characteristics and what did you notice about other team members?

How do you demonstrate your willingness to listen to the inputs and opinions of colleagues?

How does team structure impact on psychological safety?

What is your approach to resolving conflict in the team?

What skills do you have in bringing colleagues together to solve a problem?

What is your experience of highlighting how care could be improved? What structures do healthcare organisations need to have to enable staff to speak up?

What might stop you from speaking up in the workplace?

Consider your approach to supporting a colleague experiencing a personal challenge that is affecting their work.

5.5   Roles and Responsibilities

The job description and pre-interview visit will give you an opportunity to clarify the role and key responsibilities. It is important to be able to demonstrate how you will be able to meet these competencies by describing your skills and qualifications and providing examples that demonstrate your clinical and leadership abilities.

Working within a healthcare team requires an understanding of the roles and responsibilities of the other team members. When this is not well understood, it can lead to challenges such as lack of clarity during patient handover, friction within teams and disruptive behaviour. Good team leadership ensures there is clarity around responsibilities. Team members are empowered and encouraged to develop in their roles in order to contribute to the team goal. Clinical leaders should develop their emotional intelligence in order to work as effectively as possible with colleagues and patients. The reflective exercises in this chapter coach you by describing your strengths in teamwork and your understanding of what is necessary for a team to function well and in the context of the wider healthcare system.

The delivery of healthcare is rarely carried out in isolation. Organisations and regulators expect that doctors and healthcare professionals will be able to work well together in order to deliver the highest quality care in the most compassionate way possible. Colleagues have an expectation that their contributions will be respected and that they can grow in skill and confidence in the workplace. Being a modern healthcare leader provides an opportunity to both deliver care and influence how it is delivered. See Box 5.4.

Box 5.4 'Coach Approach'
Consider a recent experience of working within a team.

Did you have a clear leadership role?

How well did you understand the responsibilities of other team members?

Was there a good communication structure and regular feedback on progress?

Were team members empowered to develop their skills?

How did the team link their work to the wider organisation?

> Was there collaborative working with other teams?
>
> What was the culture within the team and did this align with organisational culture and values?
>
> How was disruptive behaviour addressed within the team?
>
> Was there a structured approach to resolving conflict within the team?

Teamwork Questions Chapter 5

- Using an example, can you tell us about your approach to teamwork in the outpatient/inpatient setting?
- Can you describe how you will assist the department to achieve service goals?
- Can you share your approach to conflict within a healthcare team?
- Tell us about your experience of working with a team to deliver a service improvement.
- Can you share your experience of working collaboratively across traditional healthcare boundaries in order to deliver better care for patients?
- Do you think emotional intelligence plays a part in healthcare outcomes?

References

1. West MA, Lyubovnikova J. Real teams or pseudo teams? The changing landscape needs a better map. Ind Org Psychol. 2012;5(1):25–8. https://doi.org/10.1111/j.1754-9434.2011.01397.x. https://onlinelibrary.wiley.com/doi/abs/10.1111/j.1754-9434.2011.01397.x
2. Hollenbeck J, et al. Beyond team types and taxonomies: a dimensional scaling conceptualization for team description. Acad Manag Rev. 2012;37(1):82–106. https://doi.org/10.5465/armr.2010.0181.

Communication in Healthcare

6

Communication is an important area in healthcare therefore it is very likely that a number of questions will incorporate facets of communication such as your personal style of communication, impact of communication in teams and adverse outcomes when communication does not go well. This chapter will highlight some useful literature and the coach approach sections will help you develop answers that demonstrate your communication skills in your interview.

Remember the competency-based *STARR* approach when structuring your examples around communication.

Situation—the context of your example, e.g. where you were working and the team

Task—what did you need to do?

Action—what clinical skills you used and how you delivered the care/intervention?

Result—what was the outcome for the patient/team?

Review—what did you learn?

C. T. Lundy, *The Medical Interview Coach*,
https://doi.org/10.1007/978-3-031-16321-0_6

6.1   Background

In the UK, the General Medical Council has a clear focus on communication in the document Duties of a Doctor (https://www.gmc-uk.org/-/media/documents/caring-for-doctors-caring-for-patients_pdf-80706341.pdf). This highlights the importance of communicating on a personal level, more strategic communication within teams and when collaborating with others in the wider health care community. This is a useful structure for any answer on communication with three memorable points.

- Personal
- Team
- Community

Good communication is essential in the healthcare environment. When it does not go well there is a recognised association with adverse events. In preparation for your interview it is important to consider your style of communication. This chapter will help you identify and describe how you communicate in different situations.

When considering personal communication with patients and their families it is recognised that a shared understanding of the healthcare issue is fundamental to good communication and facilitates appropriate management of the patient's healthcare in the years ahead. In practice, this takes place when the healthcare provider has sufficient time to really listen, to understand the patient's concerns, and can explain the issues in a way that the patient and their carers or family can understand. Often owing to time pressures medical information can be delivered in a 'briefing' style' which does not allow for the development of a mutual understanding or shared treatment plan. A compassionate approach to healthcare involves understanding the patient's difficulty and doing something to help. This is only truly possible when there is good communication.

There are a number of ways in which good communication can be encouraged:

- Consider the environment. Is it private for example?

- Have you sufficient time set aside for the consultation or meeting?
- What preparation can you do that will help, e.g. review scans or speak with other experts?
- Have you any materials such as written information, details of support groups or websites?
- Written information on treatment plans or drug information.
- Do you need another healthcare professional present, e.g. nurse specialist or pharmacist?

When communicating medical information it is worth taking as much time as possible to prepare so that you provide information in an intentional and purposeful manner. Language should be clear and as unambiguous as possible and avoid the use of acronyms and abbreviations. In line with GMC guidance communication should be open, honest and transparent.

Communicating with colleagues in the workplace should also be afforded the same respect, with a polite and considerate approach. Taking time to prepare before a team meeting or handover is helpful as the information is more likely to be pertinent and useful. Sharing medical information in handovers can be aided by the use of handover tools. You may have used specific tools such as ISBARR or IPASS. See Boxes 6.1 and 6.2.

See National Institute of Clinical Excellence (NICE) Guideline 94 March 2018 [1].

Box 6.1 ISBARR

- **Identity of the patient.**
- **Situation.**
- **Background**
- **Assessment.**
- **Recommendation.**
- **Readback—to check clarity and understanding.**

> **Box 6.2 IPASS**
> - **Illness severity.**
> - **Patient summary.**
> - **Action list.**
> - **Situational awareness.**
> - **Synthesis by receiver.**

There are a number of other communication tools that are frequently used in 'huddles' and 'handovers'. The Royal College of Physicians in the UK has some guidance on acute care handover in their practical 'Toolkit' documents (https://www.rcplondon.ac.uk/guidelines-policy/acute-care-toolkit-1-handover). The surgical operating environment has benefited from the introduction of the 'surgical safety checklist' as a means of structuring communication and ensuring that team members are all familiar with the plan for the session and the participating staff (https://www.who.int/teams/integrated-health-services/patient-safety/research/safe-surgery). For further reading, the leading surgeon and public health researcher Atul Gwande has written extensively in this area.

Barriers to communication can also occur in the healthcare environment and may contribute to adverse events. It is increasingly recognised that 'human factors' such as fatigue, hunger and decision overload can impact on how healthcare professionals communicate. Environmental factors such as an unfamiliar workplace or a new pattern of working may also have a negative impact on communication. In addition, a healthcare professional may be anxious if they are new and unfamiliar with the team. A lack of a 'shared language' in the healthcare workplace can lead to reduced understanding around a clinical situation. A rigid hierarchy may adversely affect the likelihood of staff feeling able to develop a shared understanding of a treatment plan or process. Lack of competence may also affect the ability of a healthcare worker to communicate a concern regarding a treatment plan. Personal communication style can also have an impact on patient safety and relationships with colleagues. A team member who has an open and approachable style, provides clear unambiguous instructions and regularly checks in with colleagues regarding the treatment plan and ensures good communication structures are in place to support patients and colleagues are less likely to experience difficult or challenging situations. See Boxes 6.3 and 6.4.

Box 6.3 'Coach Approach'
Using the SBARR approach consider examples of when you have had to communicate challenging or complex information to a patient or relative.
Did you use some of the strategies outlined above?
What was the outcome?
Did you receive any feedback?

Box 6.4 'Coach Approach'
Think about a situation where communication with a patient or relative did not go as well as you might have hoped.
What did you learn from this experience?
What do you do differently as a result of this?
What training or resources have helped you develop your communication skills?

Can you link your approach to the guidance on team communication recommended by regulatory bodies, for example The General Medical Council in the UK. See Box 6.5.

Box 6.5 'Coach Approach'
Think of a situation when you had to communicate with a team about a medical plan.
What was your approach in terms of preparation, structure, supporting information and checking understanding?
Did you use any communication tools or strategies?
What was the outcome?

Learning from harm is vital. A publication from NHS England (https://www.england.nhs.uk/signuptosafety/wp-content/uploads/sites/16/2015/09/su2s-comms-safety.pdf) noted that up to 70% of adverse events were related to communication. Conflict can arise when communication lacks clarity or there is a lack of shared understanding. This can be influenced by behaviour in the work-place, for example when an individual is rude or very brief in their provision of information. Strategies that assist good communica-tion and reduce the likelihood of a conflict situation arising include a focus on the values and behaviours expected in the workplace such as respect, dignity, openness, honesty, an appre-ciation of the contributions of others and a collaborative and participative approach with a focus on delivering safe, high-quality care. See Table 6.1.

Improving communication strategies in the healthcare environ-ment involves a thoughtful approach to the purpose of the com-munication. Is the purpose of the communication to explain or share information or break bad news. How intentional have you been about your preparation for a meeting or consultation, have you been able to provide resources or signposts to patient support groups for example? Is your message going to be clearly under-stood, will you have to think about how to provide information

Table 6.1 What does this look like in practice?

• Polite introductions
• Thanking individuals for their contribution
• Clear handover procedures
• Shared documentation and support materials
• Structured roles and responsibilities
• Systems for team communication
• Meetings with a structure and agenda
• Shared language regarding clinical care
• Clarity around team goals and purpose
• Regular review of adverse events and learning
• Regular review of staff and service user feedback

that is simplified or child friendly? Developing documents that are used by patients and clinical staff is another way of developing shared understanding and ensuring structures are in place to facilitate good communications within teams.

6.1.1 Chapter 6: Sample Communication Questions

Try using the STARR approach to incorporate an example into your answer for each question.

Situation—the context of your example, e.g. where you were working and the team.

Task—what did you need to do?

Action—what clinical skills you used and how you delivered the care/intervention?

Result—what was the outcome for the patient/team?

Review—what did you learn?

Can you tell us about your communication style in the workplace?

What do you think good communication looks like in a healthcare team? Can you provide an example from your practice?

Using an example, can you tell us how you ensure that you communicate well with patients and their families?

Can you share an example of how you dealt with a challenging conversation in the workplace?

What factors do you feel impact on communication in the workplace?

Have you experienced dealing with an adverse event in the health care setting? What was the approach to learning from harm?

What is your approach to managing conflict in the healthcare environment?

6.2   Your Personal Approach to Communication in the Interview

Your interview is an important 'communication event'. As part of your preparation you should reflect on your style of communication. Many healthcare interactions are very 'transactional' when it comes to communication for example during an end-of-shift handover, the most important information is exchanged in a brief style and clarified quickly. During an interview, you will need to be able to flex from this style to a more engaging 'story telling' type of communication that will allow all panel members to understand your competence and also get a sense of your approach to healthcare.

6.3   Tell Your Story

A storytelling approach is engaging and can capture the panel's attention. Think of situations where there was a particularly challenging situation. Describe the 'call to action' that was required. Were there challenges? How did you overcome them? What was the end result and how did you, the patient and your team feel along the way? You could also describe what you learnt and what the future will look like as a result.

Consider the needs of your audience. Some of the panel will not be clinical professionals and it is important to be able to provide context for your answers. Avoid criticism of colleagues when responding to questions regarding conflict or communication. The interview is a forum for assessing your abilities and approach to situations rather than a 'debrief'.

Outlining the structure for your answer at the beginning is helpful and ensures you remain focussed on your delivery. When considering the main message of each answer focus on the key points of the question and structure your response to describe your competence and experience in relation to these key points (where possible using examples). Take every opportunity to present in formal and informal situations in the months before an

Table 6.2 Interview question feedback structure

Did you engage your audience?
Were you able to set the scene in terms of clinical and organisational context?
Were the examples clear and relevant?
Did you describe key competencies and skills clearly?
Was there a reference to healthcare behaviours and values?
Were key results in terms of patient care described clearly?
Was patient confidentiality respected during the answer?
Was there a summary of the important messages?

important interview. This will build your confidence and allow you time to improve. It is also worth practicing your delivery of answers well in advance with a friend or colleague who can give you constructive feedback (See the feedback template below). See Table 6.2.

Reference

1. National Institute of clinical Excellence (NICE) Guideline 94 March 2018.

Managing Conflict in the Healthcare Environment

7

Working in healthcare involves caring for individuals at a vulnerable time in their life. This can make communication emotional and challenging. Teams can feel under enormous pressure and there can be conflict in terms of interpersonal relationships and leadership style. Resources may not be ideal and the frustration and difficulties associated with this can lead to breakdown of relationships between clinical staff and managerial or commissioning teams. We recognise all of these as part of the healthcare environment and yet the day-to-day delivery of care and the rewards with a sense of purpose and the joy of helping another human being is what encourages healthcare professionals to stay, and to work together to improve care and the working environment. This chapter provides guidance on how to coherently describe how you would manage a conflict situation in the workplace and how to share your personal experiences in a relevant, respectful and professional manner that ensures confidentiality is maintained. The STARR approach to a competency-style question can help you to structure examples that demonstrate your ability to work through a negotiation or conflict situation in a focussed way.

Situation—the context of your example, e.g. where you were working and the team.
Task—what did you need to do?

C. T. Lundy, *The Medical Interview Coach*,
https://doi.org/10.1007/978-3-031-16321-0_7

Action—what clinical skills you used and how you delivered the care/intervention?

Result—what was the outcome for the patient/team?

Review—what did you learn?

Reminder—Ensure that any example you prepare respects patient confidentiality and is respectful towards colleagues.

7.1　Background

The healthcare interview provides the panel with a chance to ask you about your approach to clinical and workplace challenges. Many organisations are keen to see the values and behaviours you will bring to the department and organisation. You can anticipate a question on conflict management or negotiation around providing a service or making a change to care delivery.

Conflict can arise when a patient or their family raises a concern about the care provided. It is essential to be able to confidently communicate how you might approach a scenario like this and use examples of how you have supported patients and your clinical team when this situation has arisen. As mentioned in the previous chapter, it is important to be thoughtful and compassionate about any description of the clinical context and the actions of others when providing an example of a situation where workplace conflict has arisen. It is also vital to respect patient confidentiality and the reputation of professional colleagues and organisations. Your answers should focus on your approach, values, behaviours and skills. It is also important to demonstrate awareness of the support available where there is a serious conflict, for example from senior management colleagues and human resources colleagues. See Box 7.1.

> **Box 7.1 'Coach Approach'**
> Consider a time when patient care fell short of expected standards.
> How was this addressed?
> Was this an adverse incident?

What organisational policies did you use to ensure correct procedures were followed to reduce the risk of any further harm?

How did you and the team communicate this to the patient or family?

How did this meet the GMC standards around open and honest communication?

Did you prepare and have information to share with them?

What supports did you offer (e.g. psychology services or patient liaison team)?

How did you communicate with the wider team about the issue (e.g. clinical leads and senior managers)?

Did you have to provide support to colleagues?

Did you need support? Counselling or a debrief?

Was the experience emotional? How did you address this (if there was anger for example)?

7.1.1   Conflict in a Healthcare Team

Conflict can occur within the team and can arise owing to external pressures or factors such as real or perceived performance issues. When preparing for an interview question in this area it can be helpful to think over times when you have witnessed or experienced conflict in the workplace between colleagues and some of the factors that might have led to the situation deteriorating.

- Fatigue.
- Workload.
- Under resourcing.
- Emotional strain.
- Moral injury (where healthcare professionals are part of a situation or system where care is delivered in a manner contrary to their values).
- Communication issues.
- Administrative problems.

These factors provide context to the situation and can help you set the scene for any example you wish to share. It is important to acknowledge that some individuals demonstrate unacceptable behaviours in the workplace that can lead to conflict such as bullying or harassing a colleague, violent or aggressive behaviour or demonstrating poor professional behaviour such as not fulfilling clinical commitments in an agreed manner. These situations should be addressed appropriately with support of professional colleagues in management and human resources in an organisation. If you have any doubts about how to manage a conflict situation it is always wise to seek support and review organisational policies that are there to provide clarity and guidance.

In preparing answers you could consider using an example. Describe how you recognised some of the factors that led to the conflict and how you were able to support colleagues in moving forward with a solution. This will provide the panel with a sense of your ability to deal with these situations in a professional, respectful and compassionate manner whilst ensuring patient safety is your first concern. See Box 7.2.

Box 7.2 'Coach Approach'
Consider a team conflict that you helped resolve.
  What was the key issue?
  Why did a team member feel upset or annoyed?
  What action did you take?
  What influenced your approach e.g. training?
  What supports did you suggest could be useful?
  How was the issue resolved?
  What did you learn?

Putting good structures in place around communication such as regular meetings about team goals and performance can help address some of the factors that spark conflict at the early stages before they become more significant and lead to team breakdown.

Share your experiences when you have seen workplace strategies that have helped prevent or de-escalate conflict.

Healthcare regulators such as the GMC in the UK (https://www.gmc-uk.org/-/media/documents/caring-for-doctors-caring-for-patients_pdf-80706341.pdf) provide clear guidance which you should review as part of your preparation. The guidance highlights the importance of good working relationships with colleagues and the need for respect in the workplace.

7.2   Challenging Conversations

Emotional healthcare situations can be very stressful and can lead to 'difficult' or challenging conversations. Some of the conflict situations you may have encountered in clinical practice may have been in the context of a very emotional or tragic situation. If you are thinking of sharing an example that involves a very emotional scenario it is important to prepare well and consider if you will be able to share the story without becoming distressed or upset during the interview. As mentioned previously it is important to respect confidentiality during the interview. There are a number of communication strategies that we can use particularly when sharing bad news with a patient or family. Brouwer et al [1] identifity some of the reasons why these conversations may not go well and how healthcare preofessionals can prepare more appropriately in their Article. The interviewers will want to hear an objective and balanced view of a clinical scenario which provides them with insight into how you are likely to deal with a similar situation in the future, transforming a challenging conversation into a productive conversation. See Box 7.3.

Box 7.3 'Coach Approach'
Using the communication approaches outlined above and the competency based model describe a scenario where you had to share difficult news for example a treatment that did not deliver the desired outcome or a time when there was a clinical difference of opinion about patient care.

Situation—the context of your example, e.g. where you were working and the team.
Task—what did you need to do?
Action—what clinical skills you used and how you delivered the care or intervention?
Result—what was the outcome for the patient or team?
Review—what did you learn?

7.3   Conflict and Negotiation

Conflict can sometimes occur in the team setting when you or others are being asked to change a model of delivery of care or resources are being reallocated or are unavailable. The COVID pandemic led to numerous situations where standard care had to be postponed owing to staffing reallocation or governmental restrictions. The need to cope with the new ways of working and the strain involved in rapid reorganisation has been felt around the world.

You may wish to share examples of times where you were able to negotiate a better outcome for your service or delivered a new, more effective model of care. Articulating your approach to this in a coherent way will provide the panel with insights into your strategic approach to change and your ability to be flexible. See Box 7.4.

Box 7.4 'Coach Approach'
Consider a time when you were involved in service change that involved negotiation, for example obtaining a new piece of equipment of negotiating for more staff or resources.

How did you prepare?
Why was your solution going to benefit patients or staff?
Who were the key stakeholders and decision makers?
Did you anticipate the responses and concerns of others?
How did you address those concerns?
What did you suggest in terms of measuring the impact of the change?
What was the outcome of the negotiation?

Sample Questions Chapter 7 Conflict in the Healthcare Environment

- Can you provide an example that demonstrates your approach to managing conflict in a healthcare team?
- Can you describe a situation where you were able to resolve conflict in the workplace? What role does the organisation have in providing support for staff when there is workplace conflict?
- What do you think are the main factors that result in conflict in the healthcare workplace?
- Describe your approach to a clinical situation when care has not been delivered in the way it should been?
- What do you see as the most common reasons for conflict in a healthcare team and using an example tell us how you might address them in order to reduce the impact of conflict on patient care and improve working relationships?
- What do you see as one of the biggest reasons for conflict with patients, how do you address this in your practice?

Reference

1. Brouwer MA, et al. Breaking bad news: what parents would like you to know. Arch Dis Childhood. 2021;106(3). https://doi.org/10.1136/archdischild-2019-318398. https://adc.bmj.com/content/106/3/276.abstract

Clinical Governance 8

Clinical governance is often seen as a 'difficult' topic for interview questions. This chapter will help you describe how clinical governance underpins the delivery of safe, reliable healthcare. Using the coach approach you will become more confident in bringing your personal experience of governance in day-to-day practice to life.

The term 'governance' refers to healthcare systems and personal processes that help deliver safe, reliable and high-quality care. You should reference clinical governance in questions related to safety and quality. Whilst we recognise it is very difficult to completely eliminate risk in the healthcare environment as care becomes increasingly complex, clinical governance brings a systems approach to learning from error, and embedding clinical practices that are known to reduce risk. Governance structures encourage clinical teams to learn together using audit and quality improvement. Good governance requires an open and transparent approach and a learning culture.

8.1 Background

It is important to be familiar with the guidance provided by national regulators, for example the General Medical Council (GMC) in 'Duties of a Doctor' as described in previous chapters (https://www.gmc-uk.org/-/media/documents/caring-for-doctors-

© The Author(s), under exclusive license to Springer Nature 77
Switzerland AG 2022
C. T. Lundy, *The Medical Interview Coach*,
https://doi.org/10.1007/978-3-031-16321-0_8

caring-for-patients_pdf-80706341.pdf). The most important duty highlighted is to make the care of your patient your first concern. Maintaining a good standard of practice in clinical care requires a focus on safety, quality and dignity of patients. Using the 'coach approach' will help you reflect on your practice and develop answers that describe how you deliver high quality care.

8.2   Important Terms That Come Up in Interview Questions

The overarching clinical governance framework is composed of what are often referred to as 'seven pillars' in the UK:

- Clinical effectiveness and research
- Audit
- Risk Management
- Education and training
- Patient and Public Involvement
- Information governance
- Staff Management

Clinical governance was defined by Donaldson and Scally in 1998 [1] as a *'system through which NHS organisations are accountable for continuously improving the quality of their services and safeguarding high standards of care by creating and environment in which excellence in clinical care will flourish'*. We can break this down into three memorable areas that impact patient care:

Responsibilities—personal and organisational
Patient and public involvement
Continuous improvement

8.3   Responsibilities

In the United Kingdom the General Medical Council (GMC) highlights the importance of personal responsibilities that impact on delivery of safe patient care. Effective communication is an essential component of partnership with patients, carers and colleagues. Healthcare regulators and advisory groups worldwide provide similar guidance, it is important to review relevant documents prior to your interview. Developing good communication skills and practices results in better patient outcomes and more effective teamwork. In the previous chapters on communication and conflict you will have reflected on your personal experiences of how poor communication impacts on patient care and how good communication can improve safety, and reduce the risk of conflict in the workplace.

It is vital to have an honest, open and transparent approach so that a learning culture can thrive and trust is present both with patients and colleagues. The GMC website is a useful resource as it highlights each of these factors and breaks them down into practical explanations of what they mean in terms of clinical practice.

Another important document related to personal responsibilities is the Seven Principles of Public Life outlined by the UK government and applies to all people working within any civil service roles such as health, education social and care services. ref.www.gov.uk   (https://www.gov.uk/government/publications/the-7-principles-of-public-life/the-7-principles-of-public-life%2D%2D2). See Box 8.1.

1. Selflessness
2. Integrity
3. Objectivity
4. Accountability
5. Openness
6. Honesty

Box 8.1 'Coach Approach'
Use the GMC website guidance as a template to reflect on times when you exhibited an open, honest and transparent approach to patient care.

How do openness and transparency impact patient safety?

Consider examples of how you have seen trust in a team setting and what that means for clinical practice. Reflect on times when you observed or experienced a lack of trust, what impact did that have and how could it have been improved?

What do you do to demonstrate accountability in your practice?

7. Leadership

8.4   Keeping Knowledge and Skills Up to Date

An important part of our personal responsibility as a healthcare professional is to ensure we are up to date and competent in our area of clinical practice. Regulators work with employers to ensure this personal aspect of 'governance' is supported by access to personal development opportunities such as training courses and conferences. It is continuously assessed through patient and colleague feedback, workplace appraisal and license-to-practice reviews. To fulfil the requirements of these processes clinicians are expected to show evidence of how professional knowledge and skills are maintained and how good, respectful working relationships with patients and colleagues are maintained.

Annual appraisal is an opportunity for practitioners to review their practice and continuous professional development. Some roles may involve appraisal duties. *You should ensure that your appraisal is up to date and any license to practice or revalidation has been processed prior to your interview if possible.*

8.5   Organisational Responsibilities

Clinical audit is an important part of governance in the NHS in the UK and many other countries. Doctors should be able to demonstrate awareness of important national clinical guidelines and relevant regulations wherever they are practicing. Organisations use clinical audits as a method of assessing if clinical care is meeting accepted standards and will help clinical staff identify areas for improvement and inform patients about service standards. Audits of practice can take place locally when a unit reviews practice against an agreed standard with the aim of learning and improving care. If you practice in the UK it is important to be aware of the active national audits in your clinical area such as the National Heart Failure Audit, National Audit of Dementia and the Paediatric Intensive Care Audit network. See Box 8.2.

Box 8.2 'Coach Approach'
Reflect on your contribution to local or national audits as a way to describe your approach to assessing standards of care delivery.

Have you undertaken a benchmarking exercise in your unit?

What national standards of care are you familiar with in relation to your area of specialist practice?

How did audit impact on care delivery in your experience?

Were patient views included and what impact did that have?

An extremely important part of organisational clinical governance systems is the processes around learning from clinical incidents, possible harm and actual harm that occurs in adverse events. Questions in this area may focus on personal experience of being part of a team learning from an adverse outcome or experience of supporting a colleague who has been involved in a clinical incident. It is important to be familiar with the assessment of risk, for example many organisations will use a 'Risk matrix' to help describe the potential or actual degree of harm.

Useful documents that can help prepare for this part of the interview include documents from the UK government such as the Berwick report 'A promise to learn a commitment to act' which describes the culture of learning in the NHS (https://assets.pub-

lishing.service.gov.uk/government/uploads/system/uploads/
attachment_data/file/226703/Berwick_Report.pdf).   Familiarise
yourself with local risk assessment tools and procedures for 'serious adverse incident' reviews.

Reports such as those highlighting the difficulties in hospitals
such as Mid-Staffordshire (https://www.gov.uk/government/pub-
lications/report-of-the-mid-staffordshire-nhs-foundation-trust-
public-inquiry) also provide useful reading prior to an interview
as they are an important reminder of the difficulties that can arise
in patient care when there is a lack of awareness of the importance
of a culture focused on safety and good teamwork. NHS England
provides numerous resources to help healthcare professionals in
terms of processes and protocols that support learning when an
incident has taken place such as the serious incident framework
(supporting learning to prevent recurrence).

There is also extensive documentation available on 'never
events' with a Care and Quality Commission report—'Opening
the door to change' (https://www.cqc.org.uk/publications/themed-
work/opening-door-change) describing how we can approach
systems to ensure that barriers to each type of never event are
truly an 'strong and systemic'. See Box 8.3.

Box 8.3 'Coach Approach'
Describe ways in which you keep your professional knowledge and skills up-to-date and ensure safe practice.

How do you assess risk, what is your understanding of
organisational approaches to risk management?

Describe your approach to ensuring patient safety.

Describe your understanding of how a team can learn
from an adverse event.

Describe supports for staff following an incident.

8.6   Supporting Colleagues

Supporting colleagues when an adverse event has taken place is
something many of us will have to do and we may have required

support ourselves when clinical care has not been of the standard we would like to deliver. This area is a common interview question, for example '*Please describe your approach to support for a doctor in training where there has been an issue with poor documentation which led to a drug error*'. The GMC good medical practice guide highlights the following areas:

- Records should be clear accurate and legible.
- Records should be made at the same time as the event or as soon as possible afterwards.
- You must maintain records that contain personal information about patients securely and in line with data protection law.
- Clinical records should include relevant clinical findings, decisions made and actions agreed, who is making the decision and agreeing the actions and the information given to patients.
- Any drugs prescribed or any investigation or treatment.
- Who is making the record and when.

Responding to a question around governance, patient safety and support of a less experienced colleague also provides an opportunity to highlight your skills of communication partnership and teamwork in teaching and supporting colleagues in training. You can describe your role in supervision and teaching. It is very important to emphasise an open and honest approach when things go wrong. If a patient has suffered any harm or distress can you describe how were you able to put matters right? For example, offer an apology, explain fully and promptly what has happened and likely short- and long-term effects. It is very important that your answers are respectful at all times about patients and colleagues and that you maintain confidentiality during your interview (https://www.gmc-uk.org/ethical-guidance/ethical-guidance-for-doctors/leadership-and-management-for-all-doctors). NHS employers may also describe the values and behaviours expected within their particular trust or healthcare institution, it is important to be knowledgeable about this as it may form the basis of questions regarding your leadership style and approach to clinical governance on a personal level.

8.7   Adverse Incident Reporting and Analysis

You should be aware of your personal and organisational responsibilities in highlighting anything that could cause harm. There are a number of reporting systems, e.g. DATIX as well as local forums such as audit meetings, clinical governance meetings and medication safety committees. When a 'Significant Adverse Event' has occurred there are usually agreed procedures to explore what happened and to identify system failings that require attention. If you have experienced these processes or have had additional training in how to analyse a significant event it is useful to consider how you would describe your experience and training. See Box 8.4.

Box 8.4 'Coach Approach'

Consider a situation where care was not delivered in the way you/or the team had planned.

- Describe how you assessed what happened.
- Why did it happen, for example human factors, systems error, communication issue?
- What action did you/or the team take to ensure patient safety?
- What went wrong and consider what went well?
- How did you assess what could be changed or agree change?
- How did you identify learning?
- How were service users involved?

Adapted from HSCBoard NI.

When further investigation in a more complex situation is needed a 'Root Cause Analysis' may be undertaken with a panel of professionals looking in detail at the events and the improvements or training required as a result. In the most significant events, an independent panel may be convened particularly if the issue is very complex and technical expertise of a specific nature would be of benefit. An important recent UK NHS document is 'A Just Culture Guide' which provides suggested ways of supporting staff who have been involved in a patient safety incident (https://www.england.nhs.uk/patient-safety/a-just-culture-guide/).   This work has been based on the review undertaken by Professor Sir Norman Williams in 2018. See Box 8.5.

It is crucial that you are familiar with processes in your current position and healthcare setting so that you can explain your understanding of how to protect patients and staff from harm and also have an awareness of the processes in the new institution if it is likely to be different, for example in a different country.

Box 8.5 'Coach Approach'
Consider your experience of local clinical governance structures in your organisation:
Have you contributed to a case review or been involved in an adverse event review?

- What supports were in place to identify the potential for harm?
- Was a risk matrix was used?
- Were specific methodologies used, e.g. Root cause analysis?
- Was it possible to identify key issues that led to the adverse event, e.g. communication or technical issues?
- Were human factors considered as part of the analysis?
- What supports were there for patients and staff?
- What was the learning for the team/organisation and how was this shared?
- Were there systems changes following the review?

When reflecting on your experiences, think about how organisational values influence the way in which the review took place in terms of honesty, openness, accountability and collective leadership? Consider the impact on patients and staff during and following the review/analysis?

Remember to respect confidentiality in preparation of any examples.

8.8   Patient and Public Involvement and Engagement

Healthcare organisations and primary care providers will have a variety of structures in place to ensure that patients and the public are involved in the design of healthcare services. This will include robust means of getting patient feedback on services and staff contributions.

It is advisable to familiarise yourself with the organisation's Annual Report before the interview. This will usually include a section on their approach to Patient and Public Involvement and Engagement (This is sometimes shortened to PPIE).

Examples of patient and public involvement include obtaining real-time feedback from patients on wards or in outpatient and clinic settings, questionnaires for carers and family members, working with focus groups when planning service change, developing links with charities that specialise in working with patients and their families. Organisations usually publish their approach to complaints and how they process them as well as how they identify compliments and areas that patients and service users rate very highly.

There are national governance structures in place in the UK, for example to ensure that patients have a voice in the healthcare system and concerns can be raised through health and social care regulatory bodies such as the General Medical Council, the Nursing and Midwifery Council and the Care and Quality Commission and Monitor. Organisations may also subscribe to platforms that allow the public to comment on care such as 'Care Opinion'.

As part of revalidation and appraisal there is an expectation that you will have feedback from both patients and colleagues. This is usually called a 360-Degree feedback exercise. See Box 8.6.

> **Box 8.6 'Coach Approach'**
> Describe your experience of patient engagement with a service improvement project, for example previous service patients and engagement with a charity focus group.
>
> Have you experience working in a unit that received compliments from patients or carers? What did they particularly value? Why do you think that was so important to them?
>
> Consider what factors might lead to a complaint from a patient, e.g. communication issues.
>
> What is your experience of obtaining patient feedback on a personal and service level?

8.9   Continuous Improvement

Learning from harm or adverse incidents through an open, transparent approach is fundamental to good clinical governance. All areas of the UK have developed improvement and innovation hubs to ensure that there is a significant focus on continuous improvement in the safety and quality of healthcare.

8.10   Benchmarking and Reviewing Clinical Practice

Benchmarking is a way of comparing practice standards with other similar or leading clinical units. It is an important component of good clinical governance and is particularly relevant should you be applying for a post in a large teaching hospital or a hospital that provides regional specialty services. If your work in primary or secondary care involves delivering procedures or treatments that involve national standards it is important to be aware that this work often requires benchmarking with other similar units or healthcare settings. There are numerous ways in which NHS organisations benchmark against each other, for example

Table 8.1 Benchmarking in healthcare

• Why did your unit undertake a benchmarking exercise?
• What standards were applied?
• How was the information gathered and shared?
• What did you learn?
• Was there change as a result?
• Was change sustained?
• How was the information shared with the wider healthcare community?
• Was patient engagement and feedback part of the process?

outcomes from intensive care are submitted nationally, morbidity and mortality data is correlated with organisations of similar size and complexity where possible. See Table 8.1.

8.10.1 Reflection

If you have been involved in any benchmarking or clinical standards comparison work you could incorporate what you learnt into a response to a question around clinical governance.

8.11 Quality Improvement

Clinicians strive for the highest quality care; however, audits and patient feedback may identify areas that could be improved. New treatment standards or national guidance may also suggest a new way of managing a condition or delivering a service. Most healthcare organisations and primary care providers have embedded 'quality improvement' methodology as a way of teams working together with patients to deliver continuous improvement. The next chapter will focus on quality improvement and innovation in healthcare, a vital component of good clinical governance. The NHS in the UK has identified the 'Model for Improvement' as a standard methodology and most organisations will have this as one of their quality improvement tools.

8.12   Human Factors that Can Impact on Patient Safety

It is well recognised that there are factors that can adversely impact on patient safety that are related to the way in which individuals are affected, for example by fatigue, stress, new environments or complex unfamiliar processes.

Recognised 'human factors' that can affect patient and staff safety:

- *Tiredness*
- *Hunger*
- *Being late*
- *Unfamiliar environment*
- *Unfamiliar team*
- *Decision fatigue*
- *Language barrier/not recognising abbreviations*
- *New procedure or process*
- *Hierarchy*
- *Stress*
- *Aggression in the workplace*

As part of clinical governance frameworks, healthcare organisations should be actively trying to put systems in place that mitigate these risks. There is a growing industry looking at 'human factors' in high-risk environments including healthcare. There are numerous resources that provide free information on how 'human factors' can impact on patient care, a few are listed below. Adverse events analysis will try and identify any human factors that could be addressed by improved systems or organisational processes. When considering how to prepare an answer about patient safety or adverse events try and include examples or experiences that highlight learning and how the team and organisation looked at the issue in the context of the system.

8.13 Answering Questions on Patent Safety and Learning from Harm

The interview is not a forum for a detailed clinical debrief and you should be mindful of this when considering your preparation of scenarios and examples you plan to share. You should respect the contribution of others and patient confidentiality. Focus on what your contribution was and what you learnt and any organisational learning. See Box 8.7.

Box 8.7 'Coach Approach'

Describe your experience of the impact of human factors on team communication for example tiredness after a long shift.

What human factors do you think are most important when a new staff member joins a team?

What organisational good practices have you seen or heard about that can reduce the risk of harm due to human factors?

What reports are you aware of that have highlighted the impact of human factors on clinical care?

Developing your answers using the reflective 'coach approach' will bring your experience of improving patient safety and reducing risk to life in the interview. Additional resources at the end of this chapter provide a further reading in this important area of clinical practice.

Sample Questions Chapter 8 Clinical Governance
- Tell us about your approach to dealing with a medical error in your unit such as inadvertent administration of the wrong medication to a patient.
- Describe your understanding of the systems in place for an adverse event review.
- How would you address the situation where a member of the clinical team has been identified as having been involved in a clinical incident involving a technical error.

- Describe your approach to managing a clinical situation where a colleague in training made a prescribing error for an inpatient under your care.
- Tell us about your understanding of systems to protect patient data and information.
- Describe your understanding of how human factors can affect patient safety if possible, using an example.
- Tell us about your experience of patient and public involvement in service improvement and co-production.
- How can we identify what is important for patient and service users in this specialty area of practice?
- What is your experience of patient feedback as a means of improving a service?

Reference

1. Scally G, et al. Clinical governance and the drive for quality improvement in the new NHS in England. BMJ. 1998;317:61. https://doi.org/10.1136/bmj.317.7150.61. (Published 04 July 1998) Cite this as: BMJ 1998;317:61

Useful Resources

https://chfg.org/what-are-clinical-human-factors/
www.mitss.org
https://qualitysafety.bmj.com/content/23/3/196
https://pubmed.ncbi.nlm.nih.gov/25077248/ (To Err is Human- Building a safer health system).
http://www.ihi.org/education/ihiopenschool/Courses/Documents/SummaryDocuments/PS%20102%20SummaryFINAL.pdf
https://www.gmc-uk.org/ethical-guidance/ethical-guidance-for-doctors/good-medical-practice
https://www.medicalcouncil.ie/news-and-publications/reports/guide-to-professional-conduct-and-ethics-for-registered-medical-practitioners-amended-.pdf
https://www.england.nhs.uk/patient-safety/a-just-culture-guide/

Improvement and Innovation in Healthcare

9

Making the care of our patients our first concern is considered one of the most important duties of a doctor. There are many opportunities to improve patient care and innovate within the healthcare environment. Medical research has delivered incredible benefits for patients. For healthcare professionals involved in research, it is important to be able to describe how this led to improvements for patients. In this chapter, you will use the 'coach approach' to work on developing clear descriptions of your efforts to improve patient care. You will learn how to develop your examples to showcase the methodologies and experience you can bring to your new role.

9.1 Background

For many healthcare professionals quality improvement work provides an everyday opportunity to improve services and patient care. The NHS in the UK has embraced a number of methodological approaches to improvement. The NHS in England encourages organisations to innovate and improve in a consistent and aligned manner. The 'Model for Improvement' developed by Edwards Deming (https://deming.org/explore/pdsa) is one approach that is now widely used in the NHS and internationally as a means of testing a change idea through iterative testing. Other

© The Author(s), under exclusive license to Springer Nature Switzerland AG 2022

C. T. Lundy, *The Medical Interview Coach*,
https://doi.org/10.1007/978-3-031-16321-0_9

UK regions have a similar approach. The NHS in Scotland, for example, has developed a national improvement strategy that has involved targeted training across health and social care sectors linked to the approach of the Institute for Healthcare Improvement in the USA. Wales and Northern Ireland have similar strategic plans in place to deliver improvement in both the quality and safety of services.

There are a number of international associations and organisations that promote quality improvement as a means of delivering better quality care including the Institute for Healthcare Improvement, Health Improvement Alliance Europe, The Q Community and The International Society for Quality in Healthcare. These bodies have similar strategic aims and provide knowledge sharing platforms and resources for healthcare professionals. They encourage a collaborative approach to improvement so that new ideas and approaches can be shared across traditional healthcare boundaries.

Healthcare professionals should be familiar with the methodology for improvement used in their own organisation. If applying to a new hospital/clinical setting it may be helpful to research the approach they take in this area of patient care, e.g. Model for Improvement, Lean / Six Sigma, process mapping, audit and national benchmarking.

A useful summary is provided at https://www.hqip.org.uk/wp-content/uploads/2021/01/Final-Quality-Improvement-QI-Tools-09-12-20.pdf

Well recognised examples of organisations that have demonstrated significant improvement in their delivery of quality care using a consistent approach include The East London Foundation Trust in England, Cincinnati Children's Hospital and Intermountain Healthcare in the USA. Intermountain, for example has championed an approach that encourages developing consistency for clinical care which aims to reduce variation in clinical practice leading to improved care and reduced cost.

Central to the development of any improvement in healthcare is the engagement with service users: what do they need from services and how can the quality and safety of care meet those needs in the most cost-effective way?

The Institute for Healthcare Improvement (IHI) developed the concept of the 'Triple Aim' *the goal of the Triple Aim is to 'improve the patient care experience, improve the health of a population, and reduce per capita health care costs'*. IHI stresses that the strategy is a single aim with three dimensions. Recently, an additional aspect has been adopted by many healthcare professionals—improved clinical experience—leading to the creation of the Quadruple Aim. The argument is that without an improved clinical experience on the provider side, the three other patient-centric aspects will not reach their full potential (http://www.ihi. org/communities/blogs/the-triple-aim-or-the-quadruple-aim-four-points-to-help-set-your-strategy).

9.2   How to Describe a Quality Improvement Project?

As an interview candidate, you should be able to provide a coherent description of how an improvement project was delivered and how improvements were sustained within the healthcare setting. A useful starting point is outlining the *vision* for the change and what the team was expected to deliver in terms of better patient care.

9.2.1   Project Aim

The next step is describing how the change project was developed including the methodology used. For example, if using the *Plan, Do, Study, Act* method of iterative testing, provide a short description of the aim of the project in terms that the interview panel will be able to understand as non-specialists in the field. It may be useful to describe the aim in terms such as 'how much', 'by when'. For example, *'The project aim was was to achieve a reduction of 50% in patients who "Did not attend" clinic X by March 2022'*.

'The benefit we hoped to deliver for patients was better access to care in a more timely fashion.

We measured this by looking at the number of new and review patients and their waiting times to be seen prior to and during the project as we tested our change ideas.'

9.2.2   Project Team

Describing the team and stakeholders involved is critical to demonstrating that the project took patients/clients views into account and that change idea were developed in a collaborative manner.

9.2.3   Stakeholders

When describing the project team consider who the significant stakeholders were in terms of delivering a successful project: patient group representatives, administrative leads, radiology colleagues and nursing colleagues. This will depend on the area of work and the interfaces that are relevant.

Clearly explain how you contributed to the project. Was there a detailed project plan and clear lines of communication within the team? If possible, describe how the project aligned to wider organisational goals or national strategies. It is also important to mention governance, the organisational sponsor highlight awareness around patient safety.

9.2.4   Project Plan

Many projects in healthcare do not succeed due to a lack of clear planning and poor use of data to measure the impact of change ideas. For any improvement project that has involved data collection, it is important to be able to describe coherently what data was collected and how it was utilised to tell the story of the project, e.g. via run charts or process control charts. The team may have been able to identify variations and any 'special cause' variations that helped understand the system better. In the interview setting it is unlikely you will need to go into great detail so it is worthwhile reviewing the key areas that your data provided guidance on in terms of project impact/improvement in care so you can be as clear and succinct as possible.

9.2.5   Measures and Outcomes

Describing outcomes in terms of the benefit for patients, safety, cost, staff and population health is the essential conclusion of your description of any improvement project. If the work has been presented or published to facilitate the 'spread' or 'scale' of the improvement project describe why this was important and how the project has gone on to deliver sustained benefits for patient care.

Being part of a team that has delivered improvements that improve safety and quality is extremely rewarding. Be enthusiastic about your achievements and share that positive experience with the panel. Include your personal learning about what contributed to the success of the project and highlight how the team overcame barriers or challenges. See Box 9.1.

Box 9.1 'Coach Approach'
Using the outline below describe an innovation or improvement project you were involved in.
Vision
Aim
Methodology
Measures
Outcomes
Ongoing work/next steps

9.3   Research and Innovation

It is easy for healthcare professionals to confuse or conflate research and quality improvement. Sometimes there is overlap between the processes. In general, however, research helps to provide answers to questions that are currently not known. Quality improvement implies that the components of good care are known with a focus on helping teams overcome barriers to delivering this.

A research protocol is usually followed rigorously once implemented. A quality improvement project is more fluid and iterative, taking into account new knowledge and ideas that are revealed as part of the process.

It is important to be able to describe the purpose and outcome of your research work in an interview. Generally, these projects involve careful planning and aim to address important clinical or population health questions. If the post has a research component it is essential to look at the output of the department and try to anticipate what questions may be asked at interview. Remember that some of the interview panel may be lay members and it is very important to be able to describe your research work in a coherent way particularly if the area is very specialised.

9.4   Describing a Research Project

As with improvement projects think about how you can articulate the question posed in a research study you took part in. *Why was this an important area in terms of patient care?*

Most research work takes place within a wider team. Prepare to describe the context of any work and the role you had especially any key areas of responsibility.

Research governance and ethical approval may come up in the interview if there is a significant research component to the post. Use examples to articulate as clearly as possible your understanding of the principles of good research governance and any ethical issues that you have faced and how your research team approached these.

Funding and publications are key metrics that you may be required to discuss at the interview. Review any funding applications you were involved in so that you can confidently and succinctly explain your role and the preparations required in successfully applying for grants as well as the financial stewardship that must follow for the duration of the project. If you have major publications that you wish to highlight at interview review, the key messages that you wish to share with the panel so that you can clearly explain the impact of the work. It is worthwhile to reflect on any unsuccessful applications or papers; could you describe your learning to the panel? See Box 9.2.

Box 9.2 'Coach Approach'
Describe a research project you were involved in using the key areas below as structure.
What question were you trying to answer…
Ethical approval
Organisational/national alignment.
Project team/Funding/Sponsor.
Timeline and management skills.
Challenges.
Training opportunities during the research—skills/techniques.
Outcomes in terms of patient benefit and for the organisation.
Ongoing work in the area.

9.5   Technology

The world of healthcare is changing at a fast rate and new technologies are resulting in significant benefits. Some of the key areas of innovation include the impact of digital healthcare, precision medicine and artificial intelligence. Consider how new technologies may impact on your field of healthcare in the coming years, what are you excited about, what do you feel is making a real difference? See Box 9.3.

Box 9.3 'Coach Approach'
Consider the topics below. Develop examples that describe relevant work you have undertaken in your field of practice that demonstrate your understanding of new technology or future approaches to delivery of care.
Patient experience and design thinking
Digital healthcare
Remote consulting
Genetics and precision medicine
Automation
Artificial Intelligence
Robotics

Try using the STARR approach to structure your answers

- *Clinical Situation*

- *Task/technology*
- *Action*
- *Result*
- *Review/learning and future applications*

Not all of these topics will be relevant to your area but it is important to challenge yourself to think outside the box during your preparation as your interviewers may be interested in trying to understand how you can contribute to the future development of the organisation.

Sample Questions: Chapter 9 Improvement, Research and Innovation
- Tell us about a service development you were involved in that delivered benefits in patient care.
- Tell us about a change that you led and describe the improvement methodology used.
- Can you describe a research project that you were involved in and tell us about the impact it had on patient care?

- What research skills will you bring to this department? Can you describe a recent project?
- Have you experienced delivering service change? Tell us how you overcame pitfalls and barriers.
- What do you think is the biggest challenge in delivering a successful research project?
- How would you take a new treatment idea forward within the department?
- What do you see as the possible areas for improvement in this speciality?
- What are the opportunities to deliver better patient care in this speciality?
- Can you tell us about a project that you were involved in that delivered an improvement in patient care?
- What technology trends do we need to be ready for in this specialty?
- Where do you see the impact of technological advances in this speciality/in healthcare?

Healthcare Education

In many healthcare roles, there is an expectation that the post holder will contribute to training undergraduate or postgraduate students. You can expect that there will be a question regarding your ability to support education and training of students and colleagues. This chapter will help you use the 'coach approach' to develop clear answers about your skills in supporting education and training. Using well-structured examples you can demonstrate your knowledge, experience and skills, providing insight into your ability to develop and support others.

10.1 Background

Modern healthcare education aims to equip professionals for lifelong learning. Many of the new undergraduate medical curricula have embraced a problem-based learning approach, following patients and their families through their healthcare journey. There may be opportunities for undergraduate students to learn in a more holistic way as they go through the various clinical placements in their undergraduate training.

Each educational placement will offer different opportunities for students to acquire new practical clinical skills. Most universities will have common threads running through curricula including communication skills, working in partnership with patients and their families, working with the wider healthcare team to

C. T. Lundy, *The Medical Interview Coach*,
https://doi.org/10.1007/978-3-031-16321-0_10

undertake investigation and management of complex healthcare conditions, research innovation and quality improvement. In the UK, the General Medical Council has provided standards that should underpin undergraduate training. There is also guidance for postgraduate training. Local deanery advisors or training coordinators can assist in clarifying the training environment and opportunities required for accreditation as a training unit.

Many primary and secondary healthcare providers in the UK work in partnership with universities to deliver a range of undergraduate teaching programmes and support postgraduate education. There are similar arrangements in other countries. This results in many permanent medical roles having time allocated for clinical and educational supervision.

You may already have substantial experience in this area and have received bespoke training in the field of medical education. There are a number of medical education postgraduate qualifications available and most UK deaneries and teaching hospitals offer regular updates such as 'teach the teacher', 'supporting the student in difficulty', 'communication skills', 'teaching for small groups' and 'teaching for large groups'.

The COVID pandemic resulted in much of the lecture-based medical education that had been delivered face-to-face being migrated onto online platforms. If you have had experience with online teaching or bespoke training in this area this might be an important area for reflection to highlight your skill set in supporting online learning. See Boxes 10.1 and 10.2.

Box 10.1 'Coach Approach'
Think about times in which you have been involved in undergraduate/postgraduate medical education:

- Have you engaged in supporting students with problem-based learning on clinical placements?
- What is your approach to supporting learning using reflective practice?

- Outline your practical experience of assisting at clinical examinations? What training have you had in providing feedback or marking? Have you experience of setting examination questions?
- Have you had training in how to support trainees who are having difficulty in progressing through training?
- What is your practical experience in working with training advisors and clinical supervisors in this situation?
- Outline specific training in simulation or particular skills such as teaching procedures, for example surgical skills, chest drain insertion and lumbar puncture.

10.2 Simulation Training

Consider if you have skills in using simulation as a means of training. Have you specific qualifications in this area? What practical experience do you have? What do you think the benefits of training using simulation?

Many healthcare providers are using simulation scenarios as means of training. It is often part of post graduate training where practical procedures or emergency scenarios allow clinicians to practice skills without risk to patients and is also used in undergraduate medical training. There is increasing demand for appropriately trained facilitators.

Box 10.2 'Coach Approach'

Do you participate in the delivery of postgraduate training courses such as advanced life support? What specific training have you received in this field? Highlight if this will bring a benefit in your new clinical role.

Have you worked specifically with university departments in the delivery of education and training for undergraduate or postgraduate students? What was your role and how did you deliver the training?

Have you been involved in delivering any interdisciplinary training (for example teaching medical students together with other disciplines, e.g. pharmacy or nursing)?

What have you learnt about different modalities of teaching as a result of your experience? What are the strengths of online learning for example? What challenges have you had to overcome in this area, for example during the COVID pandemic?

Have you received feedback on your teaching skills? What were your strengths and did you undertake any additional training as a result of the feedback?

10.3   Training Structures

It is helpful to have an understanding of the postgraduate training structure in your specialty area particularly if the job you are applying for is within a teaching hospital or primary care provider that has a training commitment. The department may already be involved in postgraduate teaching and it is likely opportunities will arise for formal education roles in time. This might be something that the interview panel is interested in even if it is not specifically listed as a component of the current role. For example, there may be an expectation that you will be able to undertake a training role such as clinical or educational supervisor role.

For many NHS hospitals and primary care providers there are requirements for doctors who have trainees working with them to undertake regular updates in education and training. Therefore, it is important to ensure this aspect of your CV is up to date prior to your interview.

10.4   Training Roles

If you have held any roles of responsibility with regards to training (for example, trainee representative working with a local training committee or Royal College in the UK in your specialty) be prepared to describe what you have undertaken as part of this role and how you think this benefited trainees and patient care. You may have been an educational supervisor or training programme director. The interview presents an opportunity for you to highlight your background in education and training and the significant skillset you can bring to the new department. Highlight the skills you learned interacting with colleagues in other hospitals and with senior leaders such as Royal College officers in developing support for trainees and your specialty or developing any courses or curriculum adjustments.

You may have undertaken specific training in quality improvement or medical leadership during postgraduate training. There are a number of fellowship programmes in many of the UK regions and in other countries such as Ireland, Australia and the USA which focus on encouraging doctors in training to learn more about leadership and management. If you have had the opportunity to undertake specific training in this field consider your experience carefully and think about what particular learning you would like to share or projects that you were involved in during your fellowship. Often these types of fellowships provide a superb opportunity to work with colleagues in management, commissioning and governmental roles. Reflect on your experiences of working with colleagues in nonclinical areas and how you would propose to apply the learning or develop these networks further in the new clinical role.

10.5   Quality Improvement Education

Quality improvement methodology has been embedded in healthcare as discussed in Chap. 9. Training others in the fundamentals of quality improvement and more advanced data analysis is becoming a significant area in healthcare education. If you have qualifications such as the Institute for Healthcare Improvement (IHI) modules or more advanced training such as a fellowship or postgraduate diploma you may feel confident in talking about how you can support quality improvement projects. If you are sufficiently skilled you may be able to support others in offering training and education opportunities. Prior to the interview reflect on your role in recent projects and your ability to lead a team, support iterative testing and use QI methodology. See Box 10.3.

> **Box 10.3 'Coach Approach'**
> What quality improvement methodologies are you most familiar with? Can you teach others?
>
> Have you developed or participated in a quality improvement project that resulted in improvements in patient care?
>
> How can your support your team in the use of data for improvement?
>
> Describe how you would communicate the impact of a proposed quality improvement project with the wider healthcare team and identify appropriate outcomes and balancing measures.

The new role may include specific responsibility for quality improvement, benchmarking and national audit. It is worth considering your training in these areas and identifying any learning needs, for example you may wish to update your quality improvement skills by undertaking a higher level training course such as a postgraduate diploma, local programmes such as Scottish Improvement Leaders or becoming part of a group such as the Q community (https://q.health.org.uk).

Many healthcare organisations also offer roles related to simulation training and human factors—it is useful to highlight any skills or qualifications you have which can support organisational learning.

10.6   Governance and Adverse Event and Structured Debrief Training

You may have received additional training in areas related to governance or management of adverse incidents, for example root cause analysis or structured debriefs which allow teams to identify environmental, human factors or systems contributors when there has been an event that has caused harm or a near miss. If you have had the opportunity to participate in departmental or organisational reviews of adverse events and are in a position to offer training to others in this field this may be an important skill to highlight during your interview.

10.7   Feedback on Your Teaching

If you have held specific education roles it is helpful to review any specific feedback that you have obtained from students and colleagues highlighting your particular style of delivery strength and any areas for development. If you have undertaken any additional training as a result of feedback or been encouraged to develop more skills in a particular area, be prepared to discuss your learning and what benefit you feel this will bring to your new role.

10.8   Research Education

Some healthcare positions have defined research responsibilities, for example many clinical oncology roles involve recruitment and support for patients during a clinical trial. There may be a specific requirement for a background in research involving a postgraduate qualification such as a PhD or Master's degree and an expectation that you have the skills to support research students. In this situation, your previous research experience, training and research output will form a key part of any interview and it is useful spending time preparing how you will describe your research training, output and approach to working within a research team and securing funding. For those who have not had the opportunity to undertake a higher degree in this area, there are short courses and postgraduate qualifications available. See Box 10.4.

Box 10.4 'Coach Approach'
Describe your research qualifications.

Describe any particular skills you have, for example laboratory-based research or qualitative research methodology. Can you train others?

What inspired you to develop skills in clinical research?

Describe projects that you have undertaken which highlight benefits for patient care.

Describe your involvement in any national or international research project and why this was important in terms of improving care in that specific field.

What have you learnt by working within a research team (for example working across disciplines and interacting with university ethics and funding bodies)?

Has your research developed your skill set in project management?

Have you led on grant applications? What did you learn from this process?

How would you describe the coproduction in research that draws patient experience and clinical research together in relation to work you have undertaken?

Are you in a position to support undergraduate or postgraduate research? Do you have any learning needs in this area?

Could you describe the importance of clinical research in your specialty area and what you anticipate will bring positive change for patients and clinicians in the next 5–10 years? Most healthcare roles have an expectation that you will be able to support training, education and research. Developing answers using the 'coach approach' in this chapter will ensure that you have the ability to share your breadth of experience with the panel and showcase your particular areas of expertise.

Sample Questions Chapter 10
- Tell us about your experience in medical education and how you can support postgraduate training in this department.
- Can you tell us how you might support a postgraduate trainee in your organisation who is experiencing challenges in completing their training, using any examples where you have supported colleagues in this way?
- Can you share your experience of research including your ability to support postgraduate students in the organisation?
- Can you tell us about your training and experience in medical education and how that might benefit this organisation?
- This department/practice is very active in research. Can you tell us how your research experience and training will benefit the team?
- What challenges have you faced in the development and delivery of a recent research project? How did you overcome these challenges?

Challenges and Opportunities

11

Working in healthcare provides a myriad of personal development opportunities. Not only do healthcare professionals learn to confront academic challenges in a focussed way but caring for patients presents daily opportunities to develop skills in evaluating treatment options, sharing information, setting goals and working with a team to ensure the best and safest care possible is delivered. The interview panel will want to get a feel for your response to pressure and how you will support and lead your team both when opportunities present themselves and when circumstances are difficult. In this chapter, you will use the 'coach approach' to develop your ability to use examples that describe challenging situations you have faced that paint a clear picture of your skills in leading a team.

11.1 Background

At times, the resources available for healthcare are not ideal and it is useful to reflect on situations when care was impacted by external factors and how these barriers were approached by you and the wider team. The COVID pandemic, for example has provided many reminders of how fragile our systems can be with shortages of critical supplies affecting healthcare around the globe.

C. T. Lundy, *The Medical Interview Coach*,
https://doi.org/10.1007/978-3-031-16321-0_11

During the pandemic or in resource-poor settings you may have experienced situations where your team had to adapt to meet challenges in a proactive way to deliver the safest care for both patients and staff. This may have involved the development of new team structures, working in new areas or delivering care remotely. Consider how you approached these situations: did your team have a clear goal for any service change that occurred and was there a sense of shared purpose? There may have been factors that helped the team identify solutions quickly. Can you describe your role in the process clearly? Simon Sinek has described the benefit of trying to get to the crux of any change in his 2011 book 'Start With Why: How Great Leaders Inspire Everyone To Take Action' [1]. See Box 11.1.

Box 11.1 'Coach Approach'
Consider a time when you overcame a challenge in the work environment…
What was the issue?
How did you feel about it?
Who was in your team?
How did you come to a solution?
What did you learn?

Approaching difficult challenges requires courage. It needs a vision that the team can work towards. A good team leader has the ability to present a clear vision and break it down into the steps or goals that will help deliver the change and ultimately lead to more effective systems. Describing why it was important to patients or staff is key to answering these kinds of questions well.

11.1.1 What Sort of Challenges Could You Describe in the Interview?

Examples could include a service having to move from a traditional face to face clinic model to one where there is a careful triage of cases that need face-to-face assessment and allocation of other consultations to a remote model such as phone or video. The vision here is both that patients referred to the service receive safe and timely intervention and that the local care provider is supported in the ongoing management. This happened in many healthcare settings during the COVID pandemic.

1.1.1   Fictional Example

Describe the challenge: A waiting time of over 6 months for a non-cancer new patient dermatology assessment.

Why this was important to patients? Many people on the waiting list may experience a worsening of their condition resulting in discomfort and anxiety. In addition, some patients may also be fearful that there is a condition such as skin cancer developing and experience reduced quality of life.

What was the vision? The team lead had a vision of improved triage leading to prompt treatment and development of a service model that could use technology to support patient care as well as build relationships with local care providers.

Change ideas included piloting a daily triage of referrals by an experienced doctor and the development of a platform where local primary care providers could send in photographs of the patient's skin alongside the background history and the treatments that had been tried.

Over a 1-month period this new model identified cases that could be optimised by the local primary care provider via guidance from the specialist, cases that had been previously known to the team and lost to follow up which could be addressed via a video or phone consultation and patients that needed a more urgent face-to-face review.

Who was involved? The team engaged with stakeholders in primary care and their hospital management structure to ensure data was collected and that the results of the pilot could be analysed to ensure there were no unintended consequences of the change in working that could adversely affect patients or staff workload or incur unexpected costs. Other key stakeholders included patients who provided feedback on their clinical assessment and local care providers who were engaged in adjusting treatment and following patients up in the longer term. Staff members recognised that they needed processes in place to ensure good governance of new ways of working including any video or phone consultation and provision of high-quality information on any treatment proposed.

What else was important in the transformational change? The environment was also a consideration and access to appropriate IT facilities such as a quiet space was required which would assist with confidentiality. Clinical and administrative staff had to undertake additional training to familiarise themselves with new systems and processes. Safety nets were agreed that if a patient or the local care provider felt that a face-to-face assessment was needed following advice or a remote consultation that this would be arranged within 4 weeks.

11.2   Outcomes

When describing any service change you should be able to clearly outline the outcomes for patients/service users and staff. These may be data-driven outcomes, for example reduced waiting times or more qualitative outcomes such as improved patient experience or improved staff engagement.

Many projects provide short-term gains in healthcare. If you have been involved in more strategic changes such as a service redesign or setting up a new model of working which resulted in sustained improvement it can be very helpful to outline to the panel the factors that you feel made the work more impactful. You may have examples of delivering healthcare in low-income countries where education, innovation and collaboration played an important role in the delivery of safe care. See Box 11.2.

> **Box 11.2 'Coach Approach'**
> Using the headings below consider projects you have been involved in that led to sustained systems change.
>
> - Alignment with strategic national or local healthcare policy.
> - Defined vision for improvement in care.

- Defined goals and outcomes.
- External and internal support for the team.
- Recognition and celebration of success.

11.3   Networks and Influencing

Approaching challenges and availing of opportunities can be difficult in isolation. Successful change is delivered when teams work together towards a shared goal. As a healthcare leader in a 'senior' position where you can effect positive change it is important to consider your role within the wider healthcare network and your ability to advocate and influence for the benefit of your patients and your colleagues. Many healthcare professionals do not take the time to really consider their network and yet it is critical to how we function day to day in the delivery of good care. See Box 11.3.

This short reflective exercise will allow you to consider your clinical and management network providing structure to questions that involve change or service development. See Box 11.4.

Box 11.3 'Coach Approach'
Can you describe your role in your current team?

Who do you report to? Do you meet regularly?

Do you interact with your senior managers to discuss service goals?

Do you spend any time with their managers? In the primary care setting do you meet with commissioning leads or attend local forums?

Have you had an opportunity to meet your service director or executive team colleagues to discuss your service or improvement ideas?

Do you link with service leads in other related disciplines (for example if you are in a surgical speciality—radiology, pathology, nursing, operating theatre managers and emergency medicine colleagues)?

Have you undertaken any collaborative interdisciplinary projects which have developed your relationships? What benefits has this provided?

> **Box 11.4 'Coach Approach'**
>
> Do you work with healthcare professionals outside your organisation? In what context, can you describe the benefits to patient care or the healthcare system?
>
> Do you have opportunities to network with colleagues in public health or commissioning roles? Can you describe the links with your clinical work and these more strategic areas of healthcare planning?
>
> Can you describe your links with national and international colleagues in your specialty area? What benefits does that bring in terms of peer support and the ability to benchmark standards of care?
>
> Do you link with colleagues in training and education roles? What impact do you have on professionals in training?
>
> Do you have any horizon scanning relationships where you have encountered new thinking and ideas in other sectors?

Taking the time to answer these questions will provide a focussed look at your networks and how you have developed them over the years and how they enhance your ability to function to the highest level in providing healthcare. The list is not intended to be exhaustive and you may have networks in other spheres such as business, politics and government. The ability to reference the power of your networks and strong relationships in your interview answers will provide the panel with a sense of the additional benefits you could bring to the department beyond direct clinical care.

11.4   Influencing in Healthcare

Delivering the best care for patients is not a static thing. Healthcare evolves daily and new interventions and ways of working can deliver improvements in quality of care. As a clinical healthcare leader part of your role will be supporting and advocating for change when required. In the previous section, you looked at your 'networks' and how they impact on the care you deliver. In this section, we will consider how you can influence within those networks.

On a personal level, some individuals will have strong communication skills and find it easy to share a vision for change, explaining why it will provide a benefit for patients and the team. Most people have to work at improving these skills over time. One of the first steps is to develop an awareness of your strengths in communication.

A leader's influence can depend on a number of factors including their emotional intelligence. One of the most significant factors in healthcare leadership is empathy. Empathy in the workplace involves the ability to listen and relate to others. It can lead to a better understanding of the challenges they face and encourage them to offer possible solutions. Really listening and connecting with others requires an ability to identify the emotions of the other individual and to pick up on nonverbal cues such as body language and facial expression. Empathic, self-aware leaders will be able to recognise distress or enthusiasm in others and connect using an appropriate tone of voice, giving time for the other person to finish what they are saying before responding. Self-aware, emotionally intelligent individuals recognise the impact of their own emotions in the workplace and self-monitor in order to regulate or adjust their own behaviour and responses to a trigger or challenge. Have you mechanisms in place to support you in managing the stresses and challenges you face in the work environment? Many healthcare professionals recognise that the increasing emotional and physical burden requires structured support such as coaching, structured physical exercise, meditation and ensuring regular breaks to rest and restore.

11.5   Reflection

Think about times when you have been approached by a colleague who wanted to share an idea or raise a concern. Consider how you responded: did you listen, did you recognise their emotions, how did this impact on your response and how did this make you feel and behave at the time? What was the outcome in the short and medium term? Looking back what have you learnt from this experience? How have you changed? Did you ask for feedback?

Maintaining curiosity and developing your self-awareness can help you improve as a member of a team and as a leader. For further reading Organisational Psychologist *Dr. Tasha Eurich's 2019 book 'Insight- How to succeed by seeing yourself clearly'*, [2] provides techniques and strategies for developing better self-awareness.

Authenticity and credibility in the eyes of your colleagues and employer can have a significant impact on your ability to influence beyond your immediate team. This is particularly relevant when responding to challenges or new opportunities. In healthcare, it is important to have a clear understanding of your professional clinical skillset and to ensure that you adhere to recommendations around maintaining your standards of practice and undertake education and training appropriate to your field. This workplace credibility is important as your team will feel more confident in a leader who is known to have high professional standards and delivers the best possible care. Demonstrating a commitment to life-long learning will encourage those around you to maintain their skills and challenge outdated practices. Clinical leaders are often involved in service change and support non-clinical managerial colleagues in describing what is required in the delivery of care. Authentic leaders demonstrate their values through their behaviour and have the ability to tell the story in a clear, meaningful way that allows the rest of the team to understand what is required and how they can help. See Box 11.5.

Leaders who have the ability to respond to workplace challenges by listening to colleagues and helping identify the relevant issues and

---

Box 11.5 'Coach Approach'
Consider a time when you were asked to assist with describing a change to patient care. This may have been a change to an individual treatment plan or something more substantial involving the wider team or system.

Reflect on why you were asked for your opinion.

What expertise did you have?

> How did you translate that into knowledge that could be shared with others?
>
> What impact did this have on patient care?

coach them to find robust solutions are the most likely to lead happy and resourceful teams. *Marissa King's book 'Social Chemistry - Decoding the Patterns of Human Connection' (2021)* [3] provides further insights into human behaviour and how our existing 'networks' can become even more productive. See Box 11.6.

> **Box 11.6 'Coach Approach'**
> Consider a situation that presented your team with a challenge, for example a complaint or setback with a patient.
>
> How did you respond?
>
> Can you describe your approach?
>
> How did you identify the main issues?
>
> Did you really listen and recognise the emotional impact on the team around you?
>
> What was your approach to identifying an appropriate response?
>
> Were you able to provide credible guidance?
>
> What was the outcome?
>
> Did you identify learning for the future and any need for change?

Responding to challenges and new opportunities also requires flexibility both personally and from the wider team. It is recognised that organisational agility is a significant factor in how well an organisation can respond to challenges. *John Kotter's 2014 book 'Accelerate (XLR8)'* [4] is a great starting point for reading more about strategic organisational agility. Some healthcare organisations are very hierarchical with process-driven operating systems which limit their ability to respond rapidly to challenges.

Where organisations have connected networks and flattened hierarchies that collaborate well towards a common goal, there is an increasingly adaptive, agile response to challenges and a better ability to seize opportunity. The COVID pandemic tested healthcare and governmental organisations ability to provide an urgent cohesive response. Many organisations found themselves working with new partners and in new areas requiring different approaches to teamwork and communication. Healthcare organisations now face a significant backlog of work which will necessitate the rapid development of strategies to deliver care as quickly and effectively as possible. It is very likely that this will form part of an interview with questions directed towards understanding your approach to developing ideas and approaches to tackling this significant workload. Prepare by reflecting on any service development you were involved in that demonstrated your team's ability to adapt to the changing needs of patients: Why was change required, was there a sense of urgency, who were the key stakeholders, were you able to demonstrate safe outcomes with new ways of working, did your team act flexibly and collaborate with other providers and clinical networks.

A doctor's ability to improve healthcare is interdependent on colleagues in the wider system. Spending some time reflecting on skills in influencing, storytelling and building successful relationships in the workplace can lead to identification of better self-awareness and areas for further personal development.

11.6   Your Personal Impact

In the previous section, we have looked at how individuals and teams respond to challenges and opportunities. Using reflective practice you can develop examples that describe your experience in responding well to the needs of your patients and your team. On a personal level, you could also use this opportunity to develop your self-awareness which could lead to improvements in your ability to demonstrate emotional intelligence in the workplace—this will have a direct impact on how you respond in the face of a challenge or opportunity. See Box 11.7.

Consider how would your teammates describe you and how would you like to be described? Your approach to challenges in

---

Box 11.7 'Coach Approach'
Consider examples or experiences you have had in the last few years where you, a mentor or senior leader have demonstrated the following character traits and personal qualities:

- *Qualities*
    - Dependable
    - Honest
    - Motivated
    - Independent
    - Creative
    - Empathetic
    - Flexible
    - Humble

- *Traits*
    - Curious
    - Empathic
    - Diligent
    - Efficient
    - Ambitious
    - Compassionate

---

the workplace will have an impact not only on patients but on your team and the wider system. Interviews are increasingly focusing on identifying how an individual is likely to respond, what behaviours and values they bring to the team and what their personal impact will be both for patients and the organisation.

Sample Questions Chapter 11

- Tell us how you overcame a significant workplace challenge?
- What do you think will have the biggest technological impact on our service area? How can we prepare for this?
- What are the most significant opportunities for improvement in this specialty area?
- Describe your experience and approach to healthcare innovation.
- How can healthcare teams work better together in overcoming workplace challenges? Can you provide an example?
- Can you describe the most influential stakeholders in service transformation in this specialty?
- Can you tell us about your experience of transformational change in the healthcare environment? What do you think influences the success of change projects in this specialty area?

After the Interview

Do not share the interview questions with other candidates—you may place yourself at a disadvantage. You should keep your own notes that will assist with future interview preparation.

If the panel asks you if you have any questions keep these brief as they may be on a tight schedule, especially if the interview is virtual. Any significant queries you have about the role should be addressed in advance during a pre-interview visit or with the recruitment team.

What if You Are Not the Successful Candidate

If you are not successful you may be placed on a waiting list. Other suitable posts may come up within the waiting list period so do consider these options when you are applying. Being on a 'reserve' list may open up other opportunities. You can ask the recruitment team about this.

It can be very helpful to obtain feedback following your interview if you have not been successful. In most organisations, the interviewers will have kept notes and interview scores may give you insight into areas where you can improve.

Any feedback should be viewed as constructive criticism that will help you develop. Reflect on the information and try to address the areas you need to work on as quickly as possible so that by the time the next interview comes around you will have made progress. It is sometimes possible to obtain verbal feedback from one of the panel members. This can be very informative especially if you feel you underperformed and could benefit from more direct feedback on your interview style or depth of answer.

Resume/Curriculum Vitae Layout

You may be asked to provide a curriculum vitae and cover letter rather than a formal application form. The letter should include a clear description of your eligibility for the role and names and contact details of your current employer and references.

Reflect on the layout of your CV, it should look professional and not distracting. Publications should be referenced in a consistent style. You should highlight your major achievements. It is useful to consider reverse date order showcasing your most recent achievements first or group by topic. The use of clear bullet points can also be easier for the reader to identify significant skills and important information rather than a narrative style.

Suggested Curriculum Vitae Layout
- Personal contact details.
- Professional qualifications including dates and awarding institutions ensure you have included any that are in the essential/desirable criteria.
- Additional qualifications.
- Membership of scientific societies/Royal Colleges with details of any position of responsibility you hold.
- Clinical skill competencies were relevant, for example surgical techniques, ability to report on diagnostic tests and specific technical skills mentioned in the essential/desirable criteria.
- Educational/research skills.
- Other areas of professional expertise.
- Publications and presentations.
- Awards/significant work-related projects.

- Employment and training starting with most recent including dates.
- Short summary of role, duties, responsibilities and notable achievements.
- Career goals.
- References and contact details.

Appendix

You may also wish to review the NHS constitution which describes services provided for people using the NHS and the NHS core values:

Working together for patients
Respect and dignity
Commitment to quality of care
Compassion
Improving lives
Everyone counts

Around the different regions of the UK, there may be adaptations of the NHS values that are important for the interview setting, however, most are broadly aligned with the values described in the NHS constitution. NHS employers may also describe the values and behaviours expected within their particular trust or healthcare institution, it is important to be knowledgeable about this as it may form the basis of questions regarding your leadership style and approach to clinical governance on a personal level. For example, the Health and Social Care system in Northern Ireland has outlined values and behaviours; working together, compassion, excellence, openness and honesty. https://www.health-ni.gov.uk/articles/progress-report-collective-leadership.

Another example is Guys and St. Thomas's NHS Foundation Trust which highlights the following values—put patients first, take pride in what we do, respect others, strive to be the best, act with integrity. NHS Scotland values are described as—care and compassion, dignity and respect, openness, honesty and responsibility, quality and teamwork. https://www.guysandstthomas.nhs.uk.

References

1. 'Start With Why: How Great Leaders Inspire Everyone To Take Action'. 2011. https://simonsinek.com/product/start-with-why/.
2. Dr Tasha Eurich 2019 'Insight – How to succeed by seeing yourself clearly'.
3. Marissa King 'Social Chemistry – Decoding the Patterns of Human Connection' (2021).
4. John Kotter 2014 'Accelerate (XLR8)'.

Further Reading

https://deming.org/explore/pdsa

http://www.ihi.org/education/IHIOpenSchool/Pages/default.aspx

https://www.gov.uk/government/publications/report-of-the-mid-staffordshire-nhs-foundation-trust-public-inquiry

https://www.gmc-uk.org/-/media/documents/caring-for-doctors-caring-for-patients_pdf-80706341.pdf

https://www.medicalcouncil.ie/news-and-publications/reports/guide-to-professional-conduct-and-ethics-for-registered-medical-practitioners-amended-.pdf

https://www.medicalboard.gov.au/codes-guidelines-policies/code-of-conduct.aspx

https://www.gmc-uk.org/ethical-guidance/ethical-guidance-for-doctors/leadership and-management-for-all-doctors

https://www.gov.uk/government/publications/the-7-principles-of-public-life/the-7-principles-of-public-life%2D%2D2

'Leadership that gets results'. Daniel Goleman. Harvard Business Review March–April 2000

Personality and Leadership: A Qualitative and Quantitative Review. Judge et al. Journal of Applied Psychology Copyright 2002 by the American Psychological Association, Inc. 2002, Vol. 87, No. 4, 765–7,800,021–9010/02/$5.00. https://doi.org/10.1037//0021-9010.87.4.765

https://www.gmc-uk.org/-/media/documents/everyday-leadership-12_12_19_pdf-83469618.pdf

Industrial and Organizational Psychology Volume 5, Issue 1 p. 25–28, Real Teams or Pseudo Teams? The Changing Landscape Needs a Better Map, MICHAEL A. WEST, JOANNE LYUBOVNIKOVA 03 February 2012. https://doi.org/10.1111/j.1754-9434.2011.01397.x; https://onlinelibrary.wiley.com/doi/abs/10.1111/j.1754-9434.2011.01397.x.

BEYOND TEAM TYPES AND TAXONOMIES: A DIMENSIONAL SCALING CONCEPTUALIZATION FOR TEAM DESCRIPTION. January 2012. The Academy of Management Review 37(1):82–106. https://doi.org/10.5465/armr.2010.0181. JOHN HOLLENBECK ET AL.

https://www.gmc-uk.org/ethical-guidance/ethical-guidance-for-doctors/good-medical-practice/duties-of-a-doctor

https://www.gmc-uk.org/ethical-guidance/ethical-guidance-for-doctors/good-medical-practice

https://zengerfolkman.com

https://www.tablegroup.com

http://www.ihi.org/education/IHIOpenSchool/resources/Pages/AudioandVideo/Amy-Edmondson-Three-Ways-to-Create-Psychological-Safety-in-Health-Care.aspx

http://www.ihi.org/resources/Pages/IHIWhitePapers/Framework-Safe-Reliable-Effective-Care.aspx

National Institute of clinical Excellence (NICE) Guideline 94 March 2018.

https://www.rcplondon.ac.uk/guidelines-policy/acute-care-toolkit-1-handover

https://www.who.int/teams/integrated-health-services/patient-safety/research/safe-surgery

https://www.england.nhs.uk/signuptosafety/wp-content/uploads/sites/16/2015/09/su2s-comms-safety.pdf

Archives of Disease in Childhood Vol 106 issue 32021, Brouwer et al. breaking bad news: what parents would like you to know-https://adc.bmj.com/content/106/3/276.abstract

https://www.health-ni.gov.uk/articles/progress-report-collective-leadership

https://www.guysandstthomas.nhs.uk

https://assets.publishing.service.gov.uk/government/uploads/system/uploads/attachment_data/file/226703/Berwick_Report.pdf

https://www.cqc.org.uk/publications/themed-work/opening-door-change

https://www.england.nhs.uk/patient-safety/a-just-culture-guide/

http://www.ihi.org/communities/blogs/the-triple-aim-or-the-quadruple-aim-four-points-to-help-set-your-strategy

Clinical governance and the drive for quality improvement in the new NHS in England *BMJ* 1998; 317. https://doi.org/10.1136/bmj.317.7150.61 (Published 04 July 1998) Cite this as: *BMJ* 1998;317:61.

Additional Resources

https://auth.leadershipacademy.nhs.uk/login?state=hKFo2SBuMnF-yaGhkcHFCdTBuRENjc3JXdmFkU1VUbWNXZ05FYaFupWxvZ2luo-3RpZNkgTURWekFtRW0xdzQycEp6X2xMdjNrbXJPNWhUSDBDMi-2jY2lk2SBzZzg5elBVSkpGVFBUYkpuQTBHbnlIVEVUcERPM3dHQQ&client=sg89zPUJJFTPTbJnA0GnyHTETpDO3wGA&protocol=oauth2&scope=openid%20name%20email%20email_verified&response_mode=query&response_type=code&redirect_uri=https%3A%2F%2Fprofile.leadershipacademy.nhs.uk%2Fauth0%2Fcallback&nonce=b2afd78f61b41b46c3ff9286eb2ca76f